PREFACE

The six years since the publication of the previous edition of the Faculty's guidance on ethics have seen considerable changes in society and the economic landscape as well as in occupational health practice. Improved communications, both actual and virtual, are serving to speed up the trend towards globalisation of business. Communities, and therefore the workforces drawn from them, are more diverse than ever before and the activities of many companies transcend not just national boundaries but also continents. 24/7 working is becoming the norm in many sectors and technological advances have allowed many people to work without the constraints of a specific location or set hours. The benefits that these changes can bring to society are balanced by new risks, both physical and psycho-social, to workers. The economic downturn has had the paradoxical effect of increasing demands on many in work while depriving many others of the opportunity to earn a living. Similarly, the pressures of an ageing population have seen working lives extended for many while youth unemployment soars.

As society becomes less homogenous the drive to increase individual autonomy grows stronger. This is reflected in a greater emphasis on human rights and the empowerment of the individual. Personal information is increasingly seen as a resource with value and one over which the data subject should have greater control. Greater knowledge and easier access to information through the internet has shifted the balance of power in professional relationships so that a paternalistic approach to the client has, to a large extent, been replaced by a guiding and advisory role. In healthcare the mantra to 'put people at the heart of care' is a manifestation of this shift and has profound implications for all practitioners. The tensions in occupational health that arise from having responsibilities to multiple parties can be heightened by these changes and a clear understanding of not just legal provisions but also the fundamental ethical principles is becoming ever more important.

Occupational health professionals have had to develop a range of new skills to help organisations deal with this rapid pace of change while themselves dealing with substantial changes in the way that they deliver services. The trend to outsource services has continued as has the increasingly multidisciplinary nature of what falls within the remit of 'occupational health'. Not only physicians and nurses but also physiotherapists, psychologists, occupational therapists and others now routinely make up the clinical team. Professional organisations are adapting to these changes but perhaps not as quickly as the issues that they can generate are emerging. It is in this context that this new edition of ethical guidance has been rebadged as being for 'occupational health practice' rather than for 'occupational physicians' as previously. The change in title is not cosmetic; the guidance has been rewritten comprehensively to try and encompass the issues faced by all working in the field of occupational health and input has been drawn from practitioners with a much wider range of backgrounds than ever before.

I welcome this new publication and I hope that it provides occupational health professionals with a useful resource to help them practise in an increasingly complex world. Inevitably the document often raises questions rather than providing simple answers because the hallmark of a professional is to think through issues and to come to a balanced judgement about the right course of action to take. It is not, and cannot be, a rule book to be followed slavishly in order to avoid criticism or sanction. It does however, address very many of the issues that occupational health professionals face on a regular basis and I believe that the guidance given is both pragmatic and wise.

Olivia Carlton
President
November 2012

N.B. available online as member of FOM (new edition — 2018).

CONTENTS

CONTENTS

CONTENTS

1 INTRODUCTION

1.1 Guidance on ethics was first published by the Faculty of Occupational Medicine in 1980, recognising the importance of shared ethical principles to underpin practice. The first edition noted that the guidelines 'may have to be revised from time to time as attitudes in society continue to change'.

Background

1.2 Ethics is the term used to describe ways of examining and understanding moral life, how we decide what is right and wrong and why we come to these conclusions. Ethics as applied to professional practice becomes a voluntary framework of guiding principles of what is and is not acceptable behaviour. It is a moral code that may drive developments in the law and it bridges the gap between legal provisions and otherwise free actions. The framework gives transparency to and helps manage society's norms and expectations; as such it is not determined by healthcare professionals and it will change over time.

1.3 There is a close relationship between ethics and the law with both governing professional practice. Ethics may be more dynamic and quicker to change than rules developed through the legislative process. The two elements tend to reflect each other but they are not necessarily identical and, indeed, may conflict. Ethical practice transcends political boundaries and, particularly in an age of globalisation, professionals need to consider how the principles should be applied in a local setting as well as complying with national laws.

Drivers for change since 2006

1.4 Since the sixth edition was published in 2006 there have been significant changes in the world of work. Many organisations now operate internationally, the rapid developments in communications technology have fostered a 24/7 culture and both outsourcing and offshoring work have become commonplace. The increased pace of change has led to requirements for workers to reskill regularly throughout their working lives and in many sectors job security has diminished. Flexibility has increased in terms of work patterns and remote working bringing both benefits to and pressures on work-life balance. The economic downturn and mass migration have impacted on the availability of work in many societies and there has been an even greater focus on business costs with increased competition in the private sector and budgetary cuts in the public sector. The health and work agenda has consequently gained greater prominence, as improved work capability, reduced sickness absence and increased productivity have been seen as central to economic success.

1.5 Within the UK there have been a number of developments that have impacted significantly on occupational health practice since the publication of the previous edition. These include new equalities legislation,[1] revised guidance from the General Medical Council (GMC) on consent and confidentiality [2-4] and Faculty of Occupational Medicine publications on good occupational medical practice[5] and standards for accreditation of occupational health services.[6] These are all referred to in more detail in relevant sections of this guidance.

Status of the guidance

1.6 This ethics guidance for occupational health practice has been approved by the Board of the Faculty of Occupational Medicine. It represents a consensus view developed principally by members of the Faculty's Ethics Committee in consultation with a range of other stakeholders. During its development input was sought from interested occupational health professionals, professional bodies representing a range of disciplines, users of occupational health services and those responsible for policy development. A list of those individuals and organisations that have contributed and been consulted is given in the Acknowledgements section at the end of the document.

1.7 The document is a statement of views at a point in time. It is recognised that circumstances may change before the next edition is published and interim guidance will be published by the Faculty if considered appropriate. It is not a legal document but it could be persuasive in, for example, an employment tribunal, as an indication of current accepted norms for ethical occupational health practice. Adherence to the guidance may also influence bodies such as the Information Commissioner that data protection requirements have been met.

Multidisciplinary occupational health practice

1.8 Previous editions of the document were presented as ethics guidance for occupational physicians. However most occupational health professionals now work in multidisciplinary teams and this is reflected in the composition of the Faculty's Ethics Committee as well as in the quality standards for occupational health organisations. Consequently, although this guidance is a publication of the Faculty of Occupational Medicine, it has been written for and by a broad range of occupational health professionals. This 7th edition has therefore been retitled *Ethics Guidance for Occupational Health Practice* to reflect both its genesis and its likely audience.

Terminology

1.9   The term **'worker'** is used throughout (with reference to former or prospective workers where relevant). This term has the widest meaning as it includes the self-employed and contract workers, and is recognised internationally. The term 'employee' is avoided as the specific legal meaning is too narrow and excludes a number of people to whom occupational health professionals will provide services.

1.10   The term **'patient'** is not used as it implies a therapeutic relationship which is not a feature of many types of occupational health contact. It is recognised that 'patient' is the term used by the UK General Medical Council (GMC) in its guidance but this document is intended for use by a range of occupational healthcare professionals (not just doctors) internationally; the advantages of maintaining consistency of terminology with the GMC are considered outweighed by the disadvantages of using this term. Neither the absence of a therapeutic relationship between an occupational physician and the worker nor the occupational physician's relationship with the employer exempts the doctor from the general duties imposed on all members of the medical profession.

1.11   The term **'therapeutic relationship'** implies a duty to treat, which is not usually the case in occupational health practice, where the intervention may have biopsychosocial benefit but often involves only assessment, facilitation and signposting. A clear distinction must be made between advising on occupational health matters and offering treatment. The service boundaries have the potential to become blurred in some organisations, particularly those employing general practitioners (GPs) in a dual role.

1.12   The term **'should'** is used when the guidance would generally apply and is the recommended, but not necessarily the only, way to carry out the activity in an ethical manner. The term **'must'** implies compulsion and is taken to mean that the recommendation is the only acceptable way to ensure that the activity is ethically appropriate.

Ethical principles and values

1.13   Ethical analysis is an ancient discipline developed in many different cultures. Although there are many ethical theories, the basis of modern biomedical ethics is a system of common values based on four main principles or shared moral beliefs. These are set out briefly below to provide some context but a detailed exposition of ethical theory and its application to medicine and healthcare is beyond the scope of this guidance.[7]

The four main principles of biomedical ethics are:
- respect for the autonomy of the individual;
- doing good (beneficence);
- doing no harm (non-maleficence);
- all individuals have equal rights and responsibilities (distributive justice).

1.14   These principles underpin the duty of care that all health professionals have, which govern ethical practice:
- foster autonomy for individuals, enabling them to make informed choices;
- act fairly and without prejudice;
- protect life and health at all times;
- maintain confidentiality, justifying trust.

1.15   The dual responsibility for occupational health professionals, to the worker and to the employer, remains fully compatible with principles governing ethical professional practice.

1.16   Respect for autonomy of an individual has been at the centre of medical ethics for decades. This is more easily seen within the traditional treatment aspect of healthcare. It is accepted that a competent adult has the right, for example, to decline treatment even where that decision may cause them serious harm or death. However it remains the professional responsibility to ensure that the individual has complex information presented in an accessible, understandable way, and sufficient time to make difficult decisions.

1.17   The principles for doing good and doing no harm extend back to the Hippocratic tradition and have been an unvarying tenet of biomedical ethics. They remain fundamental to the modern delivery of healthcare.

1.18   The concept of distributive justice involves ideas of fairness and the equitable distribution of both rights and responsibilities within society. Whenever a right is created, a corresponding duty is also imposed on someone or something. This concept allows a balance when analysing biomedical ethical issues between the rights of the individual, which are often viewed as pre-eminent in western society, and the individual's associated responsibilities.

1.19   Ethical professional practice is predicated by a set of values informed by societal norms and public expectation. The public and professionals will have their own perspectives, with the common aim of seeking to apply the right judgement in each situation.

Values include:
- personal characteristics such as honesty, courtesy, resilience;
- truthfulness;
- fairness, reasonableness;
- responsibility, keeping confidence.

In many societies, higher standards of behaviour are expected of healthcare professionals than of the general public to justify the confidence placed in them.

Standard setting

General Medical Council (GMC)

1.20   In the UK the GMC is the pre-eminent body ruling on the ethical behaviour of doctors. Other professional groups have their own governing bodies, for example the Nursing and Midwifery Council (NMC) and the Health and Care Professions Council (HCPC).

Faculty of Occupational Medicine

1.21   The UK's Faculty of Occupational Medicine (Faculty) works within the regulatory and standard-setting framework for professional medical practice, acting as an authoritative body on occupational medicine, ensuring standards of professional competence and providing guidance to enable ethical integrity. The Faculty expects the highest standards of professional behaviour and practice from its members. These standards also apply to all doctors working in occupational medicine at any level, whether or not they hold a Faculty qualification. The Faculty believes that employers, workers and others who make use of the services of occupational physicians have a right to expect high standards and a right to know what those standards are.[5]

1.22   The need for special consideration of ethical standards in occupational health practice arises because the occupational health professional plays a different role from that of other medical and healthcare specialists and general professionals. It also arises because employers and workers may be unaware of the ethical constraints under which the occupational health professional operates. These include tensions between the responsibility to individuals and respect for the interests of a company, its other workers and the public; the storage and handling of occupational health information in a predominantly non-healthcare environment; the complexity of determining fitness for work; business ethics in occupational health practice and aspects of occupational health research.

International Commission on Occupational Health (ICOH)

1.23   International focus for ethics in occupational health practice is predominantly through ICOH, a non-governmental professional society, founded in 1906, that aims to foster the scientific progress, knowledge and development of occupational health and safety in all its aspects. It is recognised by the United Nations and has close working relationships with the International Labour Organisation and the World Health Organisation. It produced its first *International Code of Ethics for Occupational Health Professionals* in 1992 and there have been regular updates since.[8]

Occupational health and the law

1.24   The law as it applies to occupational health practice is considerable, complex and varies in different jurisdictions. It is therefore neither practicable nor appropriate to attempt to produce even a comprehensive summary of the law in a document such as this and reference should be made to a standard text and online resources.[9] However it is considered helpful to address those areas where the law closely defines ethical occupational health practice or where the law poses an ethical conflict. As such, the interface between ethical and legal issues in elements of occupational health practice is considered in some detail in Section 6, Fitness for Work: the legal-ethical interface. The law considered is that of the UK but the principles discussed have wider relevance; even within the UK there are differences between the laws of the separate nations and examples given in this document refer to English law.

1.25   Whilst occupational health professionals are obliged to work within the legal framework of the relevant jurisdiction, they also have a professional duty to work ethically and this may result in tension or conflict. In these circumstances due reference should be made to ethical guidance such as this document, counsel should be sought from appropriate peers and consideration should be given to the need for more formal legal advice.

Human rights

1.26   Human rights underpin society and its ethical and legal frameworks. The *Universal Declaration of Human Rights* was one of the first actions undertaken by the United Nations and it forms the basis of internationally accepted behaviour. The *European Convention of Human Rights* is enshrined in the UK Human Rights Act 1998, which sets out people's basic rights and freedoms as balanced by the needs of society.

Using the guidance

1.27   This document is set out in five sections which cover:

- **Governance**
outlining the principles governing systems through which occupational health ensures accountability for quality. These cover company values and customer issues, leadership, professional relationships, and professional standards, including evidence-based practice and continuing professional development.

- **Information**
defining principles governing the collection and use of sensitive personal data, including confidentiality, consent, data protection and standards for clinical records, whether paper or electronic, and access and disclosure issues relevant to confidential clinical records.

- **Workplace health and wellbeing**
considering levels of occupational health intervention as:

  o primary prevention - covering health promotion, pre-employment assessment, risk control, immunisation and international assignments;

  o secondary prevention – covering health screening, health surveillance, biological monitoring, drug and alcohol testing and genetic testing;

  o tertiary rehabilitation – covering supporting sick workers, recommending adjustments, termination of employment issues and health-related pension benefits.

- **Research**
discussing the principles for ethical research to encourage and foster good occupational health research and to distinguish research requiring independent ethics committee approval from clinical audit and service evaluation.

- **Fitness for work : the legal-ethical interface**
including a more detailed discussion of the legal issues underpinning fitness to work considerations such as pre-employment health assessments, duty of care to workers in employment, fitness to join pension schemes, certification of sickness absence, assessment of sickness absence, fitness to attend disciplinary meetings and ill-health retirement.

1.28   The sections are cross-referenced where appropriate and include some practical examples to illustrate issues raised in the text. It is recommended that the guidance is initially read in its entirety to give a complete picture of the subject. It is hoped that individual issues are then addressed adequately in individual sections.

2 GOVERNANCE

Introduction

2.1   The concept of clinical governance is now well understood and accepted by healthcare professionals. In the context of the National Health Service (NHS) clinical governance has been defined as 'the system through which NHS organisations are accountable for continuously improving the quality of their services and safeguarding high standards of care, by creating an environment in which clinical excellence will flourish.[10] However, governance is a much wider concept which applies to the operation of organisations of all sizes and structures, whether in the public, the private or the third sector, in all industry sectors and across national boundaries. Publicly quoted companies in the UK are required to comply with the Corporate Governance Code,[11] which is based on the Turnbull report of 1999, or explain to investors why they have not, while similar provisions apply to businesses operating in the USA by virtue of the Sarbanes-Oxley Act.[12] The emphasis may differ but the principles are the same and the focus is on activities being undertaken in a way that promotes engagement with stakeholders, transparency, openness, due process, accountability and clear communication in a context of effectiveness and efficiency.

2.2   The underpinning message is that good governance strengthens sustainability of corporate activity and helps to promote effective business risk management. It should ensure that decisions at all levels are taken after appropriate process and consultation so that those affected are given real opportunities to influence outcomes. Good governance, in addition to strengthening business and professional decision making, should also provide a sound audit trail in the event that there are adverse consequences that require examination or investigation. Good governance therefore applies to all aspects of occupational health practice, not only clinical activity but also guidance given on the organisational aspects of health and the commercial elements of providing a service.

Company values and ethical codes

2.3   Organisations, whether in the private, public or third sectors, operate within and are influenced by the society of which they are a part. That society is increasingly complex as the workforce becomes more mobile and diverse, and cultural homogeneity is less common than it was. Many organisations have therefore felt it necessary to develop their own corporate values and some operate written ethical codes that set out guiding principles for the conduct of their business and their employees. While these vary somewhat by company, most address issues such as integrity, the misuse of power, conflict of interest and business relationships. Occupational health professionals, like other employees, will be expected to abide by such value sets or codes and they should therefore satisfy themselves that there is no conflict between their professional ethics and those of their employer.

2.4   Occupational health professionals, whether employees or independent contractors, have a further duty over and above their business colleagues to strive to influence company policies so the health and wellbeing of workers, and others affected by the activities of the organisation, are promoted. This advocacy role may particularly be required when work is undertaken in less affluent societies. Occupational health professionals should seek to ensure that good health and safety practice is followed regardless of geography. Where practicable, standards should equate to those applied in countries that have long embraced a health and safety culture. Consideration should also be given to the public health context in which companies are operating and occupational health professionals should be prepared to advise on the appropriateness of supplementing primary and secondary care for workers in some circumstances.

Leadership and management

2.5   Occupational physicians are often required to fulfil a leadership role either in the context of an occupational health team or more widely in their parent organisations as key opinion formers. The difference between professional leadership and team management is not always well understood; in essence leadership is about establishing vision and strategy while management is about implementation. Leaders need not be managers and managers may not be leaders, though the two roles are often combined. Ethical behaviour is a critical success factor for both.

2.6   Good leaders require much more than professional skills and competencies. They need to have a vision which they can communicate effectively and qualities, such as integrity and honesty, which will draw others to follow. An occupational physician is likely to have knowledge and training which is broader and sometimes deeper than that of colleagues from other disciplines. They may therefore be expected to see the wider picture for both individual and organisational issues and often to direct the approach that is taken. It is therefore important not only to articulate views in a cogent manner but also to listen to and take account of the views expressed by colleagues, giving appropriate weight to the training and experience that underpins them. Good leaders aim to gather as much evidence as is reasonable before drawing conclusions and they also seek input from all members of the team. Treating colleagues with respect but showing the courage to be decisive in the best interests of individual employees and/or the organisation as a whole is likely to influence the team view even when some members may not fully agree with the leader's conclusions. Being arrogant and dismissive of colleagues' views not only loses their respect but is also a failure in the behavioural standards expected of an occupational physician.

2.7 Managing an occupational health service requires a range of organisational, resourcing and budgetary skills that are not linked to any particular professional background. It is therefore not uncommon for management of the team to be vested in someone who is not the leader in professional matters and who is not an occupational physician. Especially when the roles are split, it is essential to have a clear understanding of the respective remits, the boundaries and the division of responsibilities. Team managers should develop a management style that suits their personality, meets the needs of their team and takes account of overall organisational culture. Specific skills need to be developed and require formal training just as much as core professional competencies. Interpersonal behaviours appropriate for a clinical setting may not be suitable for managing a colleague and individuals need to have clarity, in their own minds and in the way they communicate with others, about which role they are fulfilling. An occupational health professional has obligations which may not apply to managers from other backgrounds. In particular, there is a responsibility to ensure that resource levels and skill mix are suitable and sufficient to deliver agreed service levels and that conditions which would compromise ethical duties are not accepted.

Professional relationships

Multidisciplinary teams

2.8 Many occupational physicians work in multidisciplinary teams. Some work in teams which are purely clinical, with nurses, physiotherapists, psychologists, etc, while others work in a broader context with safety professionals, occupational hygienists, human resources professionals, etc. The qualities and values that an occupational physician should display with colleagues are set out in the Faculty of Occupational Medicine's publication *Good Occupational Medical Practice.*[5]

Clinical colleagues

2.9 Sharing information within a clinical team for the benefit of a worker's health is invariably good practice but the 'need to know' principle should be applied and it should be clear to those accessing a service that this is the unit's way of working. Most workers will readily understand the need to share information where they interact with several members of the team as part of the process of service delivery. However, they may not consider the requirements for purposes of professional supervision or clinical audit. Such activities should be clearly identified in the information given about the way a quality service needs to operate. The responsibility to inform workers may be discharged in a number of ways that are likely to be determined by practical considerations; leaflets or posters may be appropriate for a site-based service while the use of electronic media may be more appropriate for dispersed organisations. The critical point is that there is a good general understanding by those using the service of why such knowledge sharing is likely to benefit them, how it works in practice and what limitations and safeguards the organisation applies. Sharing clinical information within a wider non-clinical team, without specific consent, is likely to be ethically unacceptable.

2.10 Clinical colleagues from non-medical disciplines will have their own professional bodies to whom they are accountable and those bodies may issue ethical guidance.[13] There is good concordance between the ethical documents produced by the major healthcare professions but it is possible that nuances may be interpreted differently by people coming from different backgrounds. Differences in interpretation are more likely where there are significant deviations in cultural attitudes and/or legislative frameworks and this can be an issue for the growing number of occupational health professionals operating trans-nationally. In such circumstances, every effort should be made to discuss the issues in the context of mutual respect and to try to agree a common approach that satisfies the needs of the various health professionals and, most importantly, those to whom they are providing care. Ultimately all occupational health professionals are responsible and accountable for their own behaviour and, preferably having taken advice from peers, must make their own judgement about how to act in any given situation.

Non-clinical colleagues

2.11 The provision of a safe and healthy working environment requires multiple inputs. Occupational health professionals may well work in the same department as safety professionals, occupational hygienists and others who do not have a clinical background. As western economies have shifted from manufacturing to service industries, work organisation itself has become a major determinant of health and interaction with the human resources function has grown stronger. Sharing appropriate information with these non-clinical colleagues can generate substantial health benefits and failure to do so can constitute a culpable act of omission. However, care must be taken to safeguard confidential medical information about workers. Access to occupational health records must be restricted to clinicians with a need to see them and authorised support staff who have been adequately trained in matters of medical confidentiality and who are accountable for any breaches. Where information obtained in a clinical setting needs to be shared for use by non-clinical colleagues it should be anonymised and presented as group data. Care should be taken to ensure that sample sizes are large enough and that other identifiers do not compromise confidentiality. If there is any doubt about maintaining confidentiality, the occupational health professional should seek individual consent from the workers concerned [see paragraphs 3.5-3.7 on confidentiality].

Other clinicians

2.12   Occupational health professionals necessarily interact with other clinicians, outside the realm of occupational health, who are involved in a worker's care. The interaction may be to provide or obtain information, but increasingly it may also relate to shared care.

2.13   Many healthcare systems have primary care physicians who maintain a long-term relationship with a patient, deal with the majority of illnesses and coordinate specialist treatment – in the UK the great majority of people are registered with a general practitioner who fulfils this role. Within such a model it is likely to be beneficial to a worker for their primary care physician to be aware of work-related facts which may have a bearing on their health. Occupational health professionals should therefore keep this in mind when interacting clinically with workers and obtain consent to share information with the primary care physician when appropriate. It should not be assumed that the worker would wish information to be shared in this way and consent should be sought on each occasion unless there are exceptional reasons for making a disclosure without it.

2.14   Occupational health professionals sometimes need to obtain a greater level of clinical detail than a worker can provide or there may be a requirement to validate testimony. Requests for information from those providing clinical care to the worker or from a colleague asked for an independent opinion should be specific and relate only to the matter in hand. The request should explain the context of the enquiry so that the receiving clinician is better placed to provide information which is suitable and relevant but not excessive. Blanket requests for a complete set of records can rarely be justified in occupational health practice.

Consent for the provision of a report must be obtained from the worker in advance of a request being made and should make it clear what information is being sought. Consent should be obtained in writing and a copy should be forwarded with the request for information. The consent applies only to the time, condition and circumstances when it was obtained. In the UK, the Access to Medical Reports Act 1988[14] will normally apply. The same provisions apply to information sought or provided by telephone, email or any other media [see paragraphs 3.37-3.53 on consent].

2.15   The boundary between occupational medicine and clinical care is not always clear cut. In some situations (eg remote sites or hazardous installations) treatment services may be provided as part of occupational health. In some models of provision, services such as physiotherapy or psychological treatments may be offered to supplement what is available through primary care. The occupational health consultation itself may have a therapeutic component - particularly in mental health cases. The overriding principles are that occupational health professionals must not operate outside their area of competence, they must ensure the competence of anyone to whom they refer, and that once clinical responsibility is assumed it cannot be relinquished until handed over to an appropriate colleague. Continuity of care is important and the occupational physician must be careful not to subvert the role of the primary care physician who is generally better placed and better trained to provide general medical care for a worker. Where urgency or geographical isolation justify direct therapeutic intervention, every effort should be made, with the worker's consent, to keep the primary care physician informed. Particular care should be exercised by occupational health professionals working in the healthcare sector where the boundaries between patients, workers, colleagues and experts providing an opinion can become blurred, giving rise to ethical conflicts.

Workers' representatives

2.16   Promoting good workplace health is an important aspect of the duties of occupational health professionals. Workers' representatives (including trades unions, works councils, etc) can be valuable allies when reaching out to the workforce, either as a group or on an individual level. In the UK, employers and workers have a duty[15] to cooperate to promote health and safety at work and there are different legislative arrangements depending upon whether unions are recognised[16] or not.[17] Occupational health professionals should establish with the management of the organisation to which they are providing a service what role they are expected to play in dealing with workers' representatives. They should remember that, whether an employee of the organisation or providing a service under contract, they have a duty of confidentiality to the employer as well as to individual workers. Within those constraints, they should be open in explaining to workers' representatives the rationale for advice given in relation to the health of the workforce. Maintaining good working relationships and demonstrating the impartiality required of occupational health professionals can advance health at work and help to overcome the legitimate concerns that arise from time to time.

2.17   Individual workers sometimes ask to have a trade union representative accompany them to an occupational health consultation. Most occupational health professionals would normally accede to such a request but it is prudent to confirm oral consent after the purpose and process of the consultation have been explained, to do so again in advance of any physical examination and to be alert to any signs of distress during the interview which might be handled more appropriately in private. It is also prudent to clarify the role of the trade union representative, which is to provide support to their member rather than to act as a spokesperson.   Representatives can be helpful in clarifying points, especially with less articulate workers, and in reinforcing guidance given by an occupational health professional.

Employers' representatives

2.18   Occupational health services may be funded in various ways but in the UK employers normally pay directly either by employing occupational health professionals or by contracting with a provider. This direct commercial relationship can jeopardise both the perception and the reality of impartiality, which is a fundamental tenet of ethical practice in occupational medicine. Some employers may not understand this requirement for impartiality, which is not just an ethical requirement but also a practical necessity if the trust, and hence the cooperation, of the workforce is to be maintained.   Occupational health professionals therefore need to highlight the issue and demonstrate by their behaviour that it is practised consistently.

2.19   Occupational health professionals owe general duties to their employer and/or any organisation to which they are providing a service through a third party. Those duties vary in detail in different jurisdictions but, in general, they require the occupational health professional to apply their skills to the best of their ability, to maintain the confidentiality of company information they acquire as part of their role and to abide by lawful rules set by the employer. However, unlike most other employees, a health professional also has duties to those whom they see in a professional capacity and this can potentially lead to a conflict of interest.   Common areas of difficulty include the confidentiality of occupational health records and attempts to influence the outcome of an assessment.

2.20   Employers have a legal obligation to maintain certain health records, such as the results of health surveillance and records of exposure to hazardous substances. These records should be kept separate from clinical records so as to avoid confusion about appropriateness of access. Clinical records should be in the custody of an appropriate clinician, usually within an occupational health service, and disclosure should only be made to an employer's representative with the consent of the worker concerned. Legal departments in organisations have no greater right of access than any other representative of the employer and the same worker consent is required before disclosure. Non-clinical managers of services should not normally require access to clinical records; if there are concerns about the ability to maintain appropriate privacy in a department then managers may be asked to sign a confidentiality agreement such as that used for non-clinical support staff and to be subject to disciplinary procedures if confidence is breached. Similarly auditors of an occupational health service (as opposed to those undertaking clinical audit) should not be given access to clinical records without the subjects' consent; the information required for a service audit should be obtained from other sources even if this is administratively less convenient for the auditor. Difficulties that arise in these areas can usually be resolved by discussion and a clear explanation of the occupational health professional's ethical duty; reference to this guidance may be helpful, as may conferring with senior colleagues [see paragraphs 3.59-3.83 on disclosure].

2.21   Occupational health professionals are often engaged to provide an impartial opinion on a worker's functional capacity and any measures which might be indicated to adjust the work or rehabilitate the individual. The employer and the worker may have different aspirations for the outcome of the assessment and occupational health professionals must resist inappropriate pressures from either party to sway their objective and evidence-based judgement. Similarly an occupational health professional's report may often be the gateway to financial benefits for the worker from pension schemes, insurers, etc and this can influence behaviours. Opinions provided must be based on a suitable and sufficient assessment of health status and functional capacity.

2.22   Balancing these multiple responsibilities according to ethical principles is consistent with the injunction to 'make the care of your patient your first concern'.[18] That does not mean taking the side of the worker regardless of the circumstances but rather ensuring that clinical issues are given primacy. The key to operating ethically in this potentially contentious area of practice is the consistent application of fairness, openness and probity.

Government and representatives of other official agencies

2.23   The general presumption in democratic societies is that government and its representatives act in the best interests of the public. Unfortunately that presumption is not always true and, even when it is, specific action may not be in the best interests of an individual worker to whom the occupational health professional owes the primary duty. The same ethical principles that are set out elsewhere in this document should also be applied to dealings with officialdom. Information obtained in confidence should normally only be disclosed with suitable consent, and undue pressure from officials, even when based on expediency, should be resisted. In cases where the public interest is cited it is prudent to reflect carefully, to confer with one or more senior colleagues and to record the deliberations. The number of agencies with powers to seize documents has increased significantly in recent years and legal advice, such as that provided by the medical defence organisations, should be sought if seizure is attempted. Any court order to release records must be complied with.

The public and the media

2.24   Occupational health professionals will have access to a great deal of information relating to an organisation for which they provide services. That may just relate to the health of the workforce but may also include the effects of an organisation's products, processes and practices on the health of customers, consumers and the general public. Conflicts of interest may arise if the information provided by the organisation does not appear soundly based or accurate, or if it is not made available. The occupational health professional's responsibility as an employee or contractor may clash with concern for the public health or the environment. In such circumstances a public interest disclosure may be considered and it would be prudent to discuss the circumstances with senior colleagues and with a medical defence organisation. It would be rare to make such a disclosure without having discussed matters fully with the organisation concerned. Disclosure of this type may attract legal protection, such as that conferred in the UK by the amendments made to the Employment Rights Act by the Public Interest Disclosure Act 1998.[19] The Act covers a situation where a worker reasonably believes that there has been:

* the commission of a criminal offence;
* a failure to comply with a legal obligation;
* a miscarriage of justice;
* a danger to the health and safety of an individual;
* damage to the environment; or
* the deliberate concealment of information tending to show any of the above matters.

These provisions are currently under review and may be subject to amending legislation.

2.25   On occasions occupational health professionals may be approached by the media to comment on issues. It should be established in what capacity they are being asked to act – company representative, member of a professional body, independent expert, etc. Clearance should be obtained if being quoted as a representative of an organisation and it is prudent to agree in advance the 'line to take'. In general, information given should be limited to scientifically determined facts and evidence-based opinions. On no account should the health of individuals be discussed. Occupational health professionals should take care not to stray beyond their areas of competence and it should be remembered that dealing effectively with the media is a skill in itself for which training is available. It is unusual to be offered any form of editorial control after comments are made and editing can distort messages. Clarity and simplicity in comment are therefore indicated.

Professional standards

2.26   Occupational physicians, like all other doctors, have a personal responsibility to maintain and continuously improve their own standard of practice as well as to promote the transfer of knowledge to others. General guidance on good practice, such as that produced by the General Medical Council (GMC), is applicable and the more specific guidance on good occupational medical practice produced by the Faculty[5] should be referred to.

Evidence-based medicine

2.27   Occupational medicine is a clinical science with a strong emphasis on epidemiology and statistics in the specialist curriculum. Basing practice on sound scientific evidence should be the norm but remains hampered by a lack of high quality research in some areas.   Nevertheless the approach of formulating problems into questions, finding relevant evidence, interpreting the data, making a cogent decision and evaluating the outcome is one which should be adopted as standard. In the absence of appropriate evidence it is acceptable to follow consensus guidelines but the potential weakness of this approach should be taken into account. Occupational health professionals should, wherever practicable, aim to contribute to the knowledge base by disseminating findings from their practice, preferably by publication in peer-reviewed literature.

Guidelines, protocols and audit

2.28   Occupational health professionals should be aware of and take account of guidelines published by reputable bodies (examples include the National Institute for Health and Clinical Excellence, the American College of Occupational and Environmental Medicine, the Royal College of Physicians' Health and Work Development Unit, the Faculty of Occupational Medicine and the British Occupational Health Research Foundation) that relate to their area of practice. Within their own practice, and especially if working in a team environment, they should develop protocols based on current evidence to help ensure that quality services are delivered in a consistent way. They should undertake clinical audit against protocols to assess whether their own and colleagues' practice conforms to defined standards and, if there are weaknesses, take action to remedy them. Audit should be geared to the maintenance and improvement of clinical standards and should be kept separate from any performance management system so that there is clarity of purpose for both activities.

Continuing professional development

2.29　Lifelong learning is a hallmark of a professional and occupational health professionals should devote adequate time and resources to improving their skills and knowledge. Participation in one or more formal schemes for professional development is highly desirable and obtaining an external view of strengths and weaknesses is a valuable adjunct to reflective practice. Occupational health professionals who have leadership or management responsibilities should ensure that colleagues for whom they are responsible also have the opportunity and the encouragement to continuously improve their standards of practice. Issues such as budgetary constraints or service delivery requirements should be managed so as not to compromise essential education and training.

Teaching and training

2.30　The honorary title of 'doctor' as used by most occupational physicians originally meant 'teacher' and education remains a core function of those practising medicine. The requirement for occupational health professionals to provide information, instruction and training is not confined to workers but also encompasses management and both clinical and non-clinical members of the team. There is a particular obligation to pass on knowledge to future generations of occupational health professionals by contributing to curriculum development, academic instruction, practical training, examinations, etc. Occupational health professionals in positions of influence should encourage their organisations to support specialty training in whatever way is most practical. For those providing services, consideration should be given to the establishment of training posts and for those purchasing services, reflection should be given as to whether it is socially responsible to contract with organisations that make no contribution to the maintenance of professional expertise for the future.

Occupational health for customers

2.31　A great deal of occupational health provision is undertaken by staff who are not employees of the organisation which they serve. The relationship may be that of a contractor or sub-contractor or as the employee of a third party offering occupational health services. The commercial pressures inherent in this type of professional market can lead to particular ethical difficulties. Occupational health professionals must abide by sound principles of business and biomedical ethics in their dealings with their client organisations and each other in order to safeguard their own reputations and that of the specialty as a whole. Potential areas of difficulty include advertising, competence, competitive tendering, transfer of services, resourcing and contractual terms.

Advertising

2.32　Occupational health providers may wish to advertise their services and will seek to promote the benefits which may accrue to customers. Occupational physicians are subject to constraints such as those defined by the GMC in the UK (with the Nursing and Midwifery Council (NMC) providing guidance for those occupational health professionals with a nursing background), and in general these limit advertising to the provision of factual information about professional qualifications and services.[20] Organisations employing occupational health professionals are not restricted in the same way as individuals, but occupational health professionals should disassociate themselves from marketing hyperbole and should aim to ensure that advertising literature does not make claims which are not factual and verifiable.

Competence

2.33　Occupational health professionals should only accept or perform work, either on an individual basis or on behalf of their organisation, which they are competent to undertake. When tendering for work, occupational health professionals must assess the level of specialist occupational health skills required and provision should be made for referral to a higher level of competence when indicated. Similarly, occupational health professionals must recognise areas where expert knowledge is required (for example radiation, aviation, underwater medicine) and ensure that appropriate skills are applied in the delivery of the service. The terminology used to describe occupational health professionals should be consistent with the definitions applied by relevant professional bodies[21-23] and, in particular, health professionals lacking recognised specialist qualifications and training should not be passed off as being competent at the higher level. Services themselves should work to appropriate standards and be subject to quality accreditation, such

VIGNETTE 1 : Taking on occupational health work when another provider is in situ

Dr A worked for a large multinational provider of managed corporate health services. The chief officer (CO) of the occupational health division (who was not medically qualified) had been scheduled to deliver a keynote address at an international conference near Dr A's place of work but had been severely delayed by bad weather. At late notice Dr A had been asked to stand in for his CO and had been emailed the text of the opening speech. He was concerned about a section aimed at potential clients, who had their own occupational health services, which encouraged them to consider the services of his employer. Dr A felt this would breach medical business ethics and he called the CO to iterate his concerns.

Issues

Inducing breach of contract is unethical and would lead to legal liability for the company or individuals involved.

Professional guidance makes allowance for advertising clinical services in some circumstances.

Points to consider

How far can occupational health professionals go in targeting organisations to obtain business without breaching professional guidance?

Is there a difference between promoting your company's occupational health services at a conference and doing so bilaterally with a colleague in a potential customer company?

Is Dr A justified in considering the above business practice a moral dilemma?

---

as *Occupational Health Service Standards for Accreditation* (known as SEQOHS).[6]

Competitive tender

2.34   Competition can be a healthy stimulus to improve standards of occupational health and can bring benefits to both employers and workers. Tendering exercises should be conducted with integrity which implies not only honesty but also fair dealing and truthfulness. Competitors should not be denigrated in any way and great care should be taken not to damage their professional reputations. It is improper either to offer inducements in order to secure business or to make approaches to the staff of a competitor or existing provider in order to obtain commercial advantage; such behaviour is likely to fall foul of the Bribery Act 2010[24] in the UK and severe penalties can result for individuals and organisations. Care should be taken in offering or accepting corporate gifts or hospitality where a commercial relationship exists or might exist. Larger organisations are likely to have rules and procedures governing such activity. However, in any case, it is prudent to maintain a personal register and to avoid behaviour which could be interpreted as an inducement when contracts are due for review or out for tender.

2.35   Occupational health professionals employed by a provider to work with a particular client should not use their position to gain personal advantage by, for example, offering the same service independently at a lower rate or by disclosing commercially sensitive information to a competitor. Occupational health professionals acting as technical advisers in tender evaluations must not have a commercial relationship with any of the competitors, should declare any personal or professional interests and must advise objectively on the merits of each proposal.

Transfer of services

2.36   Any transfer of services, for whatever reason, should be conducted with courtesy and consideration. There may be issues relating to the employment status of existing staff and in the UK these are covered by the Transfer of Undertakings (Protection of Employment) Regulations 2006 (TUPE).[25] The abiding principle should be to safeguard the health, safety and welfare of those workers for whom the service is being provided. The outgoing provider should therefore make every reasonable effort to facilitate the handover and should not be obstructive to either the new provider or the customer organisation. The removal of any equipment or commercially sensitive material should be timed to minimise disruption to the ongoing service. Information relating to hazards, risks and control measures, which may be the property of the outgoing provider, should normally be handed over and any resource implications agreed in advance with the new provider and/or the customer organisation. Occupational health professionals choosing to transfer to the new provider under TUPE or similar arrangements must not be penalised or harassed in any way. Issues relating to the transfer of occupational health records are addressed in paragraphs 3.17-3.36.

Resourcing

2.37   The bulk of the expense in the delivery of any occupational health contract is likely to relate to the employment costs of the staff employed. In order to maintain profitability, particularly in the later stages of a contract term when margins may have been eroded, it can be attractive to a provider to reconfigure both skill mix and staffing levels. While such activities can be legitimate business practice, it is essential that

---

occupational health professionals providing professional leadership or managing service provision ensure that resources remain suitable and sufficient to meet the agreed needs of the client. In particular, access to accredited specialist expertise must be maintained and any personnel in training must continue to receive adequate supervision and protected training time. Occupational health professionals must recognise their duties not only to their employer and their client but also to any colleagues for whom they have professional responsibility and who may be more vulnerable to management pressure.

Contractual terms

2.38   Occupational health professionals should scrutinise carefully the wording of contracts of service or contracts for services. It is not uncommon for contracts to contain requirements which may be lawful but which are unethical, such as inappropriate access to records or disclosure of attendance at an occupational health centre.   Occupational health professionals signing such contracts place themselves in difficulty as this may constitute collusion or acquiescence, even if the professional is not identified as a signatory. Where doubt exists advice may be sought from, for example, colleagues, medical defence organisations, the Faculty of Occupational Medicine or representative bodies such as the British Medical Association.

3   INFORMATION

Introduction

3.1   The collection of sensitive personal data about workers is an inherent part of the practice of occupational health. Data collected must be processed to comply with legal requirements and to meet ethical and professional standards. The ethical considerations are the focus of this section but those are interwoven with good practice and the law. The law quoted is that of the UK but the principles apply more generally.

The legal principles that must be considered in this context include:
* Common Law Duty of Confidentiality;
* Data Protection Act 1998;[26]
* Access to Medical Reports Act 1988;[14]
* Access to Health Records Act 1990;[27]
* Article 8 of the European Convention on Human Rights[28] and the Human Rights Act 1998.[29]

3.2   Modern practice requires that patients are fully involved in decisions about their care, including occupational healthcare. This respect for the individual's autonomy requires that the worker is given appropriate information to inform decision making. This will include an explanation of the information that the occupational health professional may seek from the worker's treating clinician as well as the nature of the information which might be disclosed to the employer. Workers should understand how data about them will be handled and used.

3.3   Occupational health professionals must ensure that personal information entrusted to them is kept confidential, that any disclosure of that information is appropriate and, other than in exceptional circumstances, is not made without the worker's consent. The worker must be made aware of the potential consequences of the disclosure when consent is sought. There should be a written policy and guidance on data protection covering occupational health service activities. Workers should be informed of these provisions by appropriate means, which may include leaflets, websites, posters or inclusion in correspondence and forms where relevant.

3.4   If occupational health professionals provide therapeutic care, such as investigations, immunisations or treatment, they must ensure that workers are given suitable and sufficient information to give consent to any procedure.

Confidentiality

3.5   Almost all medical practice depends on the willingness of the patient to disclose personal and often sensitive or private information to a healthcare professional who, in turn, undertakes to treat that information as confidential. In occupational health practice the healthcare worker may be acting on behalf of a third party, such as an employer, but is still dependent on the worker being willing to disclose information. Workers will only make such disclosures if they have confidence that their privacy will be maintained.

3.6   Difficulties may arise for the occupational health professional if an employer has a poor understanding of what information they may expect to receive and what will not be disclosed. It is therefore prudent to clarify this issue before any work commences. It is helpful for all parties if occupational health policies on confidentiality and disclosure of information are promulgated widely to help develop trust and a better understanding of the professional and ethical standards which apply. Regular meetings with both employers and workers' representatives to discuss services may be helpful in fostering mutual understanding.

3.7   The ethical duties prescribed by professional bodies such as the General Medical Council (GMC), the Nursing and Midwifery Council (NMC) and the Health and Care Professions Council (HCPC) apply to occupational health professionals in the same way as they do to those in other specialties. The common law duty of confidentiality will also apply.

Protecting information

Data protection

3.8   The Data Protection Act 1998 governs health records in the UK but its provisions are similar to legislation in many other countries. It covers information relating to living subjects and applies to personal identifiable material that has been stored in such a way that data can be extracted whether records are on paper, in electronic format, card indices or microfiche. A health record is defined as any record which consists of information relating to the physical or mental health or condition of an individual, and which has been made by or on behalf of a health professional in connection with the care of that individual. A data controller must be identified, either by the employer or within the client company. Independent occupational health professionals may need to register themselves as data controllers. It is the responsibility of the data controller to notify the Information Commissioner of the holding of personal data.

Data protection principles

3.9   The Data Protection Act 1998 codifies principles for the UK but these reflect good ethical practice and apply more generally.[30]

Data must be:

1. *processed fairly and lawfully;*
2. *obtained for specific and lawful purposes;*
3. *adequate, relevant and not excessive for those purposes;*
4. *accurate and where necessary, kept up to date;*
5. *not kept for longer than is necessary;*
6. *processed in accordance with the rights of a data subject;*
7. *kept secure;*
8. *not transferred abroad unless to countries with adequate data protection laws.*

Standards in data protection

Record keeping standards and security of records

3.10   Good quality clinical records, whether paper or electronic, are vital to the practice of occupational health. Standards for record keeping should be set by individual occupational health providers but should meet the requirements of the professional bodies. Records should be used and stored in such a way as to prevent unintended disclosure. Particular care should be taken with portable electronic data storage devices. Occupational health professionals should ensure that they take appropriate advice from IT professionals and not rely solely on their own knowledge of data systems.

3.11   Examples of standards to be considered for records are:

- records should be clear, accurate, legible and with minimal abbreviations;
- each entry should be signed, dated and clearly attributable to the responsible professional;
- personal comments should be avoided;
- each page should be identified by name and date of birth as a minimum;
- records should be contemporaneous;
- any deletions/corrections should be dated and signed.

Access/audit trails

3.12   Access to occupational health clinical records should be on a 'need to know' basis. Doctors, nurses and other occupational health professionals should only access records when it is necessary to allow them to undertake their work. With increasing use of electronic records, the creation of an 'audit trail' will become the norm for monitoring access to occupational health clinical records in line with other clinical systems.

Staff and information governance

3.13   All staff working in occupational health services should have training in confidentiality and information governance. Clinical staff working in occupational health services must abide by the ethical code of their professional organisation. Non-clinical staff within the team should have training in this area and sign a confidentiality agreement as a condition of employment. External agencies requiring access to databases, for activities such as system maintenance, should also be subject to a confidentiality agreement.

Social media

3.14   The use of social media is expanding rapidly, both personally and professionally. Workers and occupational health professionals may use intranet and internet sites to communicate with friends, colleagues and customers. Increasingly organisations are exploiting the benefits of social media to facilitate internal communication and to promote their businesses externally using applications such as Facebook, Twitter and blogs.

3.15   Occupational health professionals should be aware that the same ethical and legal principles apply to new media as to traditional channels and should beware the potential for blurring boundaries between personal and professional activities. Care should be taken to avoid giving details that will allow the identity of a worker or others with whom they have a professional relationship to be determined. Defamatory or derogatory comments should not be made and it should be recognised that the laws on libel and slander apply to electronic communications. It should also be remembered that 'privacy settings' do not guarantee that information posted on the internet cannot become more widely distributed.

3.16   Occupational health professionals who use social media and identify their profession or employer should act in a manner that ensures they neither damage their own professional reputation nor that of their employer. Particular care should be taken about maintaining commercial secrecy in relation to information obtained through a professional role. The British Medical Association (BMA) has issued guidance which recommends that doctors should not accept as 'friends' on social media websites people who are present or former patients. Occupational health professionals should consider carefully before accepting as 'friends' people who may work alongside them or for whom they provide services.[31]

Occupational health records

3.17   The requirements for the storage and processing of paper records are generally well understood by occupational health professionals and policies and procedures have been developed by most organisations. However, the rapid development and integration of information technology into work and personal environments necessitates greater consideration of the ethical issues that may arise. The ethical and legal principles remain unchanged but the context and the manner in which they are applied may differ.

Security of records

3.18 **Paper records.** For paper records, areas to be considered should include:

- storing records in locked (preferably fire-resistant) filing cabinets with a secure key system;
- not leaving records on desks or on photocopiers, unattended;
- transporting records in a secure notes' carrier if removal is required (eg to external clients);
- locking records in a car boot, if they have to be left briefly, and not keeping them in a car overnight;
- putting a notes tracking system in place;
- devising a process for informing the subject if records are lost.

3.19 **Transfer of electronic data.** Encryption is used to protect the confidentiality of electronic data. There are varying levels of encryption and digital security that can be applied to data and occupational health professionals should seek specialist advice if their own knowledge is inadequate. Encryption should be appropriate for the circumstances and not become a barrier to communication. An analogy would be that letters sent by post may be marked private and confidential, double enveloped with tamper proof seal and sent by registered post or hand delivered depending upon the sensitivity of the documents contained. In the same way, levels of encryption will depend upon the content and potential impact of interception of data.

3.20 A high degree of care needs to be exercised with electronic communication. The consequences of a simple error can be much more significant than for paper communication and encryption and other security systems may not protect against these. It is far easier to compromise the confidentiality of large numbers of people than is normally the case with paper records. Other examples might include sending electronic communications to the wrong individual in an organisation where email addresses are similar or copying people to an email chain which includes information not intended for those recipients.

3.21 **Moving from paper to electronic records.** It is becoming increasingly common to transfer records from paper to electronic format. Advantages include reduced storage space, cost and ease of access or transfer. When arranging for paper files to be converted, occupational health professionals should seek suitable and sufficient technical guidance. Secure arrangements should be agreed for the transfer, storage, scanning and subsequent destruction of paper records with a clear audit trail of receipt and transfer. It is recommended that paper

records are retained for an agreed period before destruction to ensure any errors are identified. The digitisation process should be in a format that cannot be edited with an audit trail of the creation of files.

3.22 **Access rights.** Paper occupational health records must be held confidentially and be accessed only by members of the occupational health team on a need-to-know basis. The same principles apply equally to electronic records. Larger occupational health services may have in-house IT staff who manage the occupational health database but others will need to seek external support. Whether employed or contracted, systems administrators must be fully briefed and trained on the confidential status of occupational health records and should sign confidentiality agreements. When setting up access rights to an occupational health database with the systems administrator it is important to provide explicit written details of the requirements for access. The occupational health professional retains professional and ethical responsibility for maintaining the confidentiality of records even when there is a professional data controller.

3.23 **Converting speech to text.** New technology allows speech to be converted into an electronic voice file for further manual conversion to text or directly into electronic text. This may reduce administration costs and delays but the author of the data must take reasonable steps to ensure the accuracy of the final version, particularly where speech is being converted directly to text. Care should also be taken with telecommunications technology that converts voicemail to text since information is more easily disclosable.

3.24 **Information sent overseas for conversion to electronic data.** Data may be processed lawfully anywhere within the European Union (EU) under the provisions of the Data Protection Act. For countries outside the EU it is not always possible to secure the same level of data protection and the consent of the data subject is generally required. Occupational health professionals should endeavour to ensure that equivalent levels of data security are applied to information for which they have responsibility regardless of geography.

Retention of records

3.25 Health records created to comply with statutory requirements must be kept for specified periods, for example:

- Control of Substances Hazardous to Health (COSHH) Regulations 2002 - 40 years;[32]
- Ionising Radiations Regulations 1999 - 50 years.[33]

3.26 The retention period for clinical records is not specified in the Data Protection Act and practice varies widely. Data controllers are required to justify the retention period which they set in their policies and to destroy data for which they no longer have a legitimate use in accordance with the fifth data protection principle. *(not kept for longer than is necessary).*

3.27   The physical storage of paper records can pose a significant problem for occupational health providers in terms of space and cost. These issues are less marked for electronic records, although the selective destruction of individual records may pose some difficulties. In providing advice on retention periods occupational health professionals should consider the delayed nature of many occupational diseases and the potential value of records to both the worker and the employer. Records can also provide valuable information for future epidemiological studies and the Data Protection Act provides that personal data which are processed only for research purposes may be kept indefinitely.

Destruction of records including electronic data

3.28   Paper records must be destroyed effectively (eg shredding or pulverisation) and not disposed of in normal waste.   Occupational health professionals should ensure that appropriate standards for confidentiality are stipulated to any external provider undertaking the work. Similarly, when electronic data are destroyed expert advice should be sought to ensure destruction is effective and adequate safeguards with respect to confidentiality are applied. Simple deletion of files is inadequate and the occupational health service must seek expert IT advice to ensure that records are completely destroyed.

Ownership of records

3.29   For in-house providers of occupational health services, the employer owns the notes, paper and filing cabinet but the contents are the intellectual property of the occupational health authors. Similarly, for electronic records, the hardware and software programmes are the property of the employer, but the data held within them are the intellectual property of the professionals creating them.   Therefore the contents cannot be accessed by the employer or their agents, other than the occupational health department, without the consent of the data subject.

3.30   Occupational health records generated and held by outsourced providers or contractors will normally remain the property of the occupational health service unless alternative contractual arrangements have been made.

Transfer of records

3.31   In general terms it is good practice and in the interests of the employer and worker for occupational health records to be transferred between providers when a service is handed over. There is however no specific legal requirement to transfer records and arrangements should be agreed between the parties concerned. The data controller for the outgoing service should ensure that records are only transferred to competent persons (normally occupational health professionals) or the subjects of the data.

3.32   ***Where a company changes its occupational health provider*** (either in-house or outsourced) it is generally in the best interests of all parties for records to be transferred to the incoming occupational health provider. Workers should be notified of the transfer to a new provider and be given the option to 'opt out' of the scheme but specific individual consent to transfer will generally be impractical unless the workforce is very

---

VIGNETTE 2 : Transfer of records between providers
Dr B learned that the electronics company for whom she worked had been successful in a recent take-over of another manufacturer. After discussions with her senior manager she approached her counterpart to investigate the nature of the other company's occupational health records. There were over nine hundred sets of paper records and duplicate statutory health records. Following detailed negotiations with the relevant officers in the other company an agreement was reached concerning the proper transfer of records.
Issues
The costs involved in records transfer can be significant and occupational health providers should factor these into contract negotiations.
Distinguish carefully between clinical and statutory health records – the treatment will be different.
Processes should be kept as simple as possible – provided adequate information is given to workers and the option to opt out offered, consent to transfer can otherwise be implied.
Points to consider
What should happen to the records of employees who were deceased or had left the company?
Where is the appropriate location for statutory health records which are not medical in confidence?
Can the outgoing provider refuse to transfer occupational health records – and if so is there any action needed?

small. Consultation with workers' representatives (eg trades unions) is a common method of communicating this activity. It is the responsibility of the existing occupational health provider to ensure that this duty is discharged. Some records, for example relating to hazard control, may have commercial secrecy considerations and outgoing providers must maintain confidentiality in this respect as well as in relation to personal records.

3.33   The practical aspects of transferring records between providers of off-site services is more challenging than transferring records held on the employer's premises. Records of which files have been transferred should be made as an audit trail and an appropriate secure method of transfer must be utilised. The outgoing provider may make a reasonable charge to cover the costs associated with the transfer of records.

3.34   If the worker declines transfer of his/her records, there are various options. If the records are not required for retention by statute:
- the records can be offered to the worker to retain;
- the records can be offered to the general practitioner (GP) to retain (with consent);
- the records may be destroyed according to the process outlined above. Alternatively, the records can be retained by the outgoing occupational health provider (but a storage charge may be applied).

3.35   ***Where an organisation (employer or occupational health provider) closes down***, records not required for retention by statute may be dealt with as above. If the employer is closing down, the occupational health provider may retain the records for an appropriate period of time but it is likely that this service would not be remunerated. If the occupational health provider ceases to trade the records could, with consent or opt out, be transferred to another occupational health organisation.

3.36   ***Where a worker changes job*** it is unusual for records to transfer. Even if the new occupational health provider is the same as the provider for his previous employment, it cannot be assumed that the worker will want records to transfer. In some circumstances (eg a move within the National Health Service (NHS)) it may be in the best interests of the worker and the employer to transfer notes but specific consent should be sought from the worker affected.

Consent

3.37   Consent is a process whereby an individual, having been provided with full information and understanding the consequences, agrees to a proposed action. Consent may be implied or express.

Implied consent may apply to situations where a worker's behaviour can clearly imply that consent is given, for example holding out their arm for venesection. However, implied consent should not be relied upon except in circumstances where it is obvious, routine and generally accepted.

Express consent may be given orally or in writing. Oral consent should be documented contemporaneously in the worker's record. When obtaining consent for the release of information to an employer, express consent in writing should be obtained. According to the GMC 2008 guidance on consent:

'You should get written consent if: There may be significant consequences for the patient's employment, social or personal life'.

It is prudent to record the key elements of the explanatory discussion you have with the worker on the consent form or in the medical record; this may be achieved by using standard text.

3.38   Consent:
- is a continuous process;
- is for the purpose for which it is given;
- can be withdrawn.

3.39   A widely drawn or blanket form of consent is ethically unacceptable; for example, seeking consent to allow an occupational health professional to write to any doctor about any matter cannot be 'informed' and is therefore unacceptable. Consent should be obtained for each significant step in the process of an occupational health assessment. For example, consent for an occupational health professional to obtain a report from a GP does not constitute valid consent for disclosure of information so obtained to management or others. When obtaining consent the worker's wishes to have another person involved in the discussion (eg relative or advocate) should be accommodated.

Capacity

3.40   Under the Mental Capacity Act 2005, a person is assumed to have capacity unless proved otherwise. The GMC advises that, when obtaining consent, consideration should be given to whether an individual has the capacity to give consent: are they able to retain, use and weigh up information needed in order to make a decision? In occupational health practice it is unusual that a worker would lack capacity but consideration should be given to vulnerable workers, such as those with neurological damage, learning difficulties or who are very young. In general it can be presumed that most young people of 16 and over have the capacity to make decisions and a person should not be treated as lacking capacity because he makes an unwise decision.[34]

Consent for treatment

3.41   Consent must be obtained before examining a worker or undertaking investigations, including screening tests. Where such procedures are delegated to other staff, the occupational health professional must ensure that those undertaking the task have adequate knowledge and training and work within guidance. Occupational health professionals do not normally deliver treatment but where they do, including the delivery of vaccination programmes, appropriate consent must be obtained.[35]

Human Tissue Act 2004

3.42   Undertaking investigations using human tissue requires specific consent. When the individual lacks capacity to consent, investigations may be undertaken if the testing is primarily of benefit to that person and necessary for their treatment. If obtaining clinical information through testing which may be primarily of benefit to a third party, express consent must have been obtained from the person whose tissue is being tested. Consent can be sought from relatives following the death of a person, but impact on the relatives must be taken into account. Difficulties may arise following 'needlestick' injuries where the source patient may be unconscious or deceased and an injured healthcare worker may have to undergo treatment with post-exposure prophylaxis for possible HIV infection because the source patient's status cannot be assessed. Consultation about this particular situation is ongoing but at this point, there is no exception to the need for consent to test source patient samples.[36] Additionally this may apply to genetic testing [see paragraphs 4.33-4.37].

Consent for the preparation and release of an occupational health report

Reports to which this applies

3.43   The term 'occupational health report' in this context means the written output of a health assessment by an occupational health professional for employment purposes based on confidential information provided by the worker or, with appropriate consent, a fellow health professional. Reports based solely on information provided to an occupational health professional by the commissioning body (employer, pension scheme, insurance company, etc) are not included in this context since they do not involve disclosure of further information and simply represent interpretation of data.

Consent process

3.44   It is the duty of the occupational health professional to ensure that the subject of the health assessment has been properly informed at the outset about its purpose, its nature and its outputs, including likely consequences. The occupational health professional should ensure that the worker has consented to the process including the preparation and release of an occupational health report. Where practicable the individual's written consent should be obtained but if not (eg with telephone conversations), recording oral consent contemporaneously in the occupational health record will suffice. Consent may be withdrawn at any stage of the process but occupational health professionals do not need to obtain confirmation of consent at each stage or to remind workers of their right to withdraw. Occupational health professionals may clarify a report or give general advice to management or human resources about a condition but no further disclosure of confidential information can be made without seeking refreshed consent from the worker.

Principle of 'no surprises'

3.45   The overriding principle which occupational health professionals should apply in producing reports is one of 'no surprises'. An individual participating in an occupational health assessment should be absolutely clear about the process in which they are engaging and what will be reported about them to a third party (employer, insurer, pension scheme, occupational health provider, etc). Explanations should be given in a way that the worker is likely to understand and deliberate omission in describing the outcome of an assessment is ethically unacceptable. The most transparent method of avoiding surprises is to explain the content of the report during a consultation and to offer to show the worker a copy before sending it to the recipient.

3.46   This approach underpins the current GMC guidance on consent which prescribes a greater level of process detail than previously in relation to the release of reports for employment purposes. In particular paragraph 34 states that a doctor should:

'offer to show your patient, or give them a copy of, any report you write about them for employment or insurance purposes before it is sent unless:

i.   *they have already indicated that they do not wish to see it;*
ii.   *disclosure would be likely to cause serious harm to the patient or anyone else;*
iii. *disclosure would be likely to reveal information about another person who does not consent.'*

3.47   This level of prescription is easier to achieve with a face to face consultation in a traditional site-based service than with some of the newer service delivery models. However, the ethical principle of 'no surprises' stands regardless of the practical means by which it is discharged and occupational health practitioners should ensure that innovation in service delivery is not allowed to compromise fundamental tenets of professional practice. Copying all reports to workers as a routine when sending them out is in line with the principle of 'no surprises' and should be encouraged as good practice.

Where the worker asks to see the report before it is sent

3.48   Although many workers will not wish to see an advance copy of a report it is important to seek to understand the nature of any concerns that they may have if they do. Such concerns may often relate to perceptions of the employer's actions in response to the advice given rather than the report itself. Signposting the worker to sources of advice (eg trade union, Citizens Advice, etc) may therefore be helpful.

3.49   Simple procedures should be put in place to provide an advance copy of a report when such access is requested. A reasonable time period should be allowed between providing the report to the worker and sending it to the commissioning body; timescales should be made clear to all parties concerned. Determining what constitutes a 'reasonable' period will depend on a number of factors, such as the method used to convey the information (eg by hand, electronically, by post, etc). There should be an expectation that the worker will have received the report and had an opportunity to raise any concerns before it is passed on; in general that should be achievable within days rather than weeks. The worker should be clear how to contact the occupational health professional if they wish to comment on the contents or withdraw consent. However, there is no requirement to obtain positive affirmation that consent remains valid and introducing excessive time delays to the process is likely to be to the detriment of the worker and the employer. Where the worker highlights factual errors in the report the occupational health professional should review the impact (if any) of these errors on the judgment provided but it should be made clear to the worker and the commissioning body that professional opinions given will not be altered as a result of lobbying. Workers should also be advised that in some cases, such as where there is a legal requirement or a public interest justification, disclosure may be made without their consent.

Withdrawal of consent

3.50   Consent may be withdrawn at any stage of the process but there are potential consequences for both the worker and the commissioning body relating to withdrawal of consent for report release. Such concerns centre particularly on health assessments for safety critical roles and key occupational groups like the Armed Forces. It is important to be explicit with the commissioning body that consent may be withdrawn at any time. The occupational health professional should remind workers that if consent is withdrawn the employer will have to act on whatever information is available to them and that this may not be in the best interests of the worker. Where consent to release a

report is withdrawn, a copy should be retained within the occupational health record, clearly marked that consent has been withdrawn and that it has not been and will not be released.

Recording consultations

3.51   Audiovisual recordings may be made in certain situations in occupational health practice and consent should always be sought in advance. They are primarily for teaching and training purposes. It should be made explicit why the recording is being made, what will happen to the data, including who will have access to it, and how it will be stored. There should be a clear reason for undertaking recording and the same is true in situations where workers may seek to record a consultation for their own purposes. Steps should be taken to ensure that recordings made under such circumstances cannot be edited.

Covert surveillance

3.52   Courts have held that covert video surveillance is lawful and can be used in evidence where there is reasonable suspicion that a worker is not telling the truth about his medical condition. The Regulation of Investigatory Powers Act 2000 does not apply to such surveillance where it is undertaken by an employer investigating a case of sickness absence or an application for an ill-health retirement pension. However occupational health professionals should not be involved in the commissioning of covert surveillance because, by implication, the activity is being undertaken in the absence of consent.

3.53   Those who undertake medico-legal work may be asked to comment on surveillance and should ensure they are competent to undertake such work. Occupational health professionals should be cautious about commenting on evidence presented as they may not be aware of how the information was obtained. Those reviewing surveillance data must ensure that they comment on the facts presented and do not disclose personal data about the case. If the worker has been assessed and a report based on covert surveillance is subsequently requested, then consent is required unless comment is restricted to confirming the identity of the individual concerned. However, if a worker has not previously been seen, consent need not be sought because there can be no issues of disclosure. Further information is available in GMC guidance.[37-38]

Access and disclosure

Access to records by worker (data subject access)

3.54   The data subject has the right to access all clinical records held about him on application. The

---

VIGNETTE 3 : A case of covert surveillance

Dr C received a management referral concerning a 45-year-old male construction worker with a lengthy ongoing spell of certified sickness absence relating to low back pain. Dr C saw the worker and noted the presence of severe symptoms but a total absence of signs. Following the consultation the manager sent Dr C video recordings which were claimed to show the worker undertaking heavy manual labour at his home throughout the period of sickness absence. There was no indication that the worker had been told about the recordings. Dr C was asked whether the video evidence changed the opinion he expressed in his first report.

Issues

If, during the original consultation, the worker admitted to Dr C that he was able to carry out heavy manual labour activities at home and Dr C omitted to tell the employer, then he would be colluding with the worker in deceiving the employer.

It is ethically acceptable for an occupational health professional who has not previously been involved in the fitness to work assessment to be asked to comment on the compatibility of a medical report (including occupational health, specialist and GP reports) and video evidence obtained by management by covert surveillance.

An occupational health professional must obtain the consent of the worker to report on any video obtained by covert surveillance if there is already a relationship between them arising from a previous occupational health assessment and report.

Points to consider

What should Dr C advise the manager in this case?

In this example, will Dr C need to seek the worker's consent to any part of his subsequent actions?

Do occupational health professionals have a role in checking the veracity of a worker's story?

---

occupational health provider may withhold access if disclosure may reveal information about a third party other than another health professional or may cause serious harm to the physical or mental health of the data subject or another person. Requests should be made in writing and the occupational health provider who holds the records should respond within 40 days. A charge may be made for this as specified within the Data Protection Act.

3.55   Should the data subject challenge the information held, factual inaccuracies may be corrected but opinions given form part of the record and cannot be changed. A statement from the data subject may be attached to the record detailing their challenge.

3.56   If disclosures are to be made under the Data Protection Act about the physical or mental health of a subject and the data controller is not a health professional, then the request should be dealt with by a health professional and clinical data released to the data subject or applicant directly by the health professional and not via the data controller. If the data controller is also a health professional, this is not required.

Access to Health Records Act 1990

3.57   The provisions of this Act have largely been superseded by the Data Protection Act 1998 and the 1990 Act now only applies to medical records of deceased individuals. Third party access to the medical

records of deceased patients may be made under the provisions of the Act. Only the executor or administrator of the deceased, or a person having a legal claim arising from the death, are entitled to access.

Access to Medical Reports Act 1988

3.58   The Access to Medical Reports Act gives an individual the right to see medical reports prepared by a doctor responsible for their clinical care for employment or insurance purposes. There has long been contention around whether or not occupational physicians provide clinical care and under what circumstances the Act may apply to occupational health reports. The GMC Guidance on Confidentiality issued in October 2009 to a great extent ended the need for this debate. Occupational physicians are now advised by GMC guidance to offer an individual the opportunity to see their report before it is sent to the employer. The Data Protection Act allows subsequent access to the record including reports [see paragraphs 3.37-3.53]. Although the Access to Medical Reports Act, and indeed GMC guidance, only applies to registered medical professionals, it is good practice for any health professional producing reports for these purposes to follow the principles.

Disclosure

3.59   Disclosure of the contents of confidential clinical records can be made:

- where the worker has given their consent for the disclosure;
- where the worker has not given consent but:
  - o disclosure is required by law;
  - o disclosure is in the public interest and can be justified without consent.

Disclosure of confidential information with consent

Disclosure to employers

3.60   This is an area of practice where difficulties can arise. The GMC requirement to 'keep disclosures to the minimum necessary when considering disclosure to a third party', is crucial to occupational health practice. The employer rarely needs clinical information about an employee or applicant for employment and the occupational health professional can give all the necessary information, including recommending adjustments for compliance with the disability provisions of the Equality Act 2010,[1] without disclosing clinical information.

3.61   Where disclosure of clinical information is essential this must only be with the consent of the worker, with exceptions as above. If consent to disclose information is withheld, the fact that the consent has been withheld may be reported to the employer and does not itself constitute a breach of confidentiality. Where information provided by a third party (eg medical certificates, referral letters) gives clinical information,

even if the worker may have been the source of that information (eg the worker has told their manager about their illness), the occupational health professional should not confirm such details without the worker's consent.

3.62   In order to avoid misunderstandings over the status of information provided for occupational health purposes, documents which form part of the occupational health record should be marked as confidential to the occupational health service. This includes documents issued by the employer, such as pre-employment screening forms, which request health information and which are intended to be processed by occupational health.   Following a court decision, employers may have a right of access to medical information provided on forms if it is not explicit that the form will be treated as confidential to the occupational health service.[39] Occupational health professionals are advised not to cooperate with systems of work where medical information is sought but not handled in accordance with normal ethical rules which the individual might expect.

Statutory health surveillance

3.63   Health surveillance may be required for some workers determined by their work exposures and associated risk assessments.   Examples of regulations requiring health surveillance include:
- Management   of Health and Safety at Work Regulations 1999;[40]

VIGNETTE 4 : A difficult disclosure
Dr D was an occupational physician in a provider that supplied occupational health sessions to a local education authority. In response to a routine management referral concerning sickness absence, an infant school teacher, Mrs E, attended an appointment. She volunteered two concerns: firstly that she had not fully answered all the questions on her pre-placement employment questionnaire and secondly that she might pose a risk to the children in her care.
In her late teens Mrs E had contracted HIV. Whilst she had not been unwell at the time, the infection had been discovered during antenatal tests. Mrs E gave permission for the doctor to write to her GP and specialist. The outcome of these enquiries revealed that with treatment she had a high CD4 count and the viral count was negative. Mrs E's recent spells of sickness absence were believed to be due to side effects from the HIV drugs and time-limited minor infections.
Issues
Responsible occupational health professionals should be dispassionate in their consideration of patients' past lifestyles and seek to apply sound risk management on a case-by-case basis.
Workers have a duty to complete pre-placement employment questionnaires truthfully, though not as a general rule to volunteer information which is not specifically requested. Questionnaires should only seek information sufficient for the purpose of risk assessment for the job.
Points to consider
What should Dr D advise Mrs E concerning the omission on her pre-placement form?
Would the advice differ if her current medical status posed a risk to the children in her care?
What should Dr D include in his occupational health report in response to the management referral?

- Control of Substances Hazardous to Health Regulations 2002;[32]
- Control of Noise at Work Regulations 2005;[41]
- Control of Vibration at Work Regulations 2005;[42]
- Control of Lead at Work Regulations 2002;[43]
- Control of Asbestos Regulations 2006;[44]
- Ionising Radiations Regulations 1999;[33]
- Diving at Work Regulations 1997;[45]
- Work in Compressed Air Regulations 1996.[46]

3.64   The employer is required to hold a Health Record for these individuals, which should include only information about their fitness for work and participation in health surveillance. This record is not an occupational health document and it should not be held by occupational health professionals.   Employers and workers may require assistance in understanding this distinction.   Occupational health professionals must obtain consent from the worker for the process of undertaking health surveillance and for the results to be passed on to the employer [see paragraph 4.29].

Sharing of information to protect workforce

3.65   Information gathered through occupational health practice may affect the health and safety of individual workers within an organisation. Legislation empowers safety representatives to access anonymised information about the health of the workforce held in relation to such matters. The sharing of information in this way will help ensure health and safety objectives are met and that the workforce is protected. Data may only be shared on an individual basis if consent to disclosure is obtained and occupational health professionals must ensure that coercion is not applied. Clear agreement should be reached between employers and workers (including safety representatives where appropriate) over sharing information.

Disclosure of information to others

3.66   The consent of the worker should be obtained before sensitive personal information is to be disclosed to others, whether professionally qualified or not, including solicitors, insurers and their agents, managers or trade union representatives. Consent should also be sought when disclosure is requested by the authorities (including the Health and Safety Executive (HSE)), except when disclosure is ordered by a judge or presiding officer of a court.

Solicitors

3.67   Solicitors act on behalf of their clients but it remains good ethical practice to obtain consent for disclosure of records. It may not always be clear whether a solicitor is acting on behalf of a worker or another party and it is imprudent to rely exclusively on a consent provided by others. An example of a 'Release of Health Records' form can be found on the BMA website; this is a form prepared by the BMA and Law Society and meets

appropriate consent requirements.[47] Individuals may not realise that health issues unrelated to the case they are pursuing can be included in their records and occupational health professionals should clarify with them what they wish to disclose – all, some or just the information relating to the issue. This qualified consent can be over-ruled by a formal court order. Court or tribunal orders can be obtained for the production of occupational health records at an early stage in legal proceedings, even though the occupational health provider is not party to the action.

3.68   Individual litigants or their solicitors may authorise only partial disclosure to other relevant parties, refusing to allow release of relevant parts of the records, for example previous audiograms in a case of hearing loss that demonstrate damage unrelated to the worker's employment at the defendant's premises. In such cases, the occupational health professional should advise both parties that full relevant disclosure should be made to both sides. The solicitors should be left to agree or to obtain a court order.

3.69   Reports commissioned by a solicitor or his client at a time when legal proceedings are reasonably in prospect may be protected by legal professional privilege. They must be kept confidential and not disclosed to other parties without the consent of the commissioning solicitor or client. It would be usual for the solicitor to arrange for disclosure. The occupational health professional has a duty not to disclose to another party without consent from the individual or his solicitor, unless ordered to do so by the court. If other parties request disclosure, the commissioning solicitor should be advised, so they can take steps to prevent access. It is good practice that such medico-legal reports are not stored with the occupational health clinical records to prevent accidental disclosure. This guidance applies equally to employment tribunals.

Auditors

3.70   Recent emphasis on improving standards in occupational health provision and the need to meet accreditation standards for various organisations may result in requests for internal and external auditors to access clinical health records.   It is unethical for occupational health professionals to allow auditors to access clinical records without consent. Workers should be advised that their data may be used for this purpose and auditors should follow appropriate processes of confidentiality and disclosure. Information should be anonymised or coded wherever practicable. Where auditors require access to clinical records or non-anonymised data, they must first obtain the express consent of the individual concerned.

Disclosure of anonymised data

3.71   Anonymised clinical data may be used to protect and promote the health of the workforce

---

VIGNETTE 5 : Occupational health responsibilities in data protection

Dr F was an occupational physician in a large provider that supplied occupational health sessions to local authority councils. In response to a request under the Freedom of Information Act the data controller of a large county council had requested detailed information concerning cases of sickness absence, including work location and demographic data, in a cohort of council workers.

Dr F reviewed those data held in the electronic occupational health information system and discovered that it would indeed be possible to extract precisely the sort of information that had been requested. However, she also recognised that due to the way in which work records were organised it would also be possible for certain individual employees at some work locations to be identified. She advised the data controller of a significant risk of breaching the Data Protection Act 1998 due to the release of sensitive individual health information.

Issues

Requests under the Freedom of Information Act need to be carefully considered. It is usually unethical to release information identifying individuals, unless justified by overriding public interest.

The effort and expense required to produce the information in a format compatible with data protection principles should not be disproportionate, requiring judgement on how best to comply with a valid request.

Sickness absence records obtained through GP 'fit notes' and self-certification are not confidential occupational health records but under the control of human resources, although still sensitive personal data.

Points to consider

In this situation, what can Dr F do to meet the Freedom of Information Act request?

What information held by occupational health providers would be considered sensitive personal and health data?

---

through health and safety actions, audit or research. Workers should be clearly informed that their data may be used in this way and they should be given the option to decline the use of their data. Any research using identifiable data will require express consent and to have gained appropriate ethical approval [see Section 5, Occupational Health Research].

3.72   Requests for information under the Freedom of Information Act (FOIA), which applies in the public sector only, are becoming more frequent. Section 38 of the FOIA allows exemption from disclosure if to do so would endanger the physical or mental health or the safety of an individual. Specific information about an individual is outside the scope of the FOIA and is considered personal data to which the Data Protection Act applies.

Disclosure of confidential information without consent

Disclosure by law

3.73   Disclosure can be ordered by a judge or presiding officer of a court using a court order. It is important to check that the order specifies occupational health clinical records. An order requiring personnel records does not include occupational health clinical records. Coroners' courts have the power to order disclosure of occupational health clinical records. In normal circumstances the required documents should be produced. However, exceptionally, court orders can

be appealed if, for example, the basis on which the court asked for the information was flawed. However non-release of information subject to a valid court order is contempt of court.

3.74   A whole range of other public bodies have powers relating to the disclosure of information. Occupational health professionals should uphold their ethical duties and make sure that consent is provided wherever possible. If authorities insist on proceeding without consent, advice should be sought from bodies such as the medical defence organisations. The guidance given below is indicative and does not obviate the requirement to seek professional advice.

3.75   The police can apply to a county court judge for disclosure of medical records. A search warrant issued by a magistrate is insufficient authority.[48] Any request for information by solicitors in the absence of a court order is also insufficient authority.

3.76   The HSE has rights under the Health & Safety at Work etc Act 1974 to require disclosure of some information to perform their statutory function.[15]

3.77   Statutory requirements for the disclosure of clinical information include the need to notify certain infectious diseases.[49]

3.78   The GMC under the Medical Act 1983 can require disclosure relevant to the discharge of its fitness to

---

practise proceedings.[50]   Similar powers to order the disclosure of information have been conferred on the Health Service Ombudsman and the Care Quality Commission.

3.79   The National Health Service Act 2006 gives power to the NHS Counter Fraud Service to issue a notice to produce NHS records (including occupational health records) to detect and prosecute fraud.[51] Approval to use these powers can be sought by asking the Ethics and Confidentiality Committee of the National Information Governance Board to consider the case.[52]

3.80   There is no unified legal system in the UK and occupational health professionals should ensure that they understand and/or take suitable advice relating to the legal system that applies in a particular case. The same guidance applies to those practising in other jurisdictions where requirements may deviate even more substantially.

In the public interest
3.81   The duty not to disclose confidential information without consent is not absolute. The GMC and the NMC permit the disclosure of such information 'in the public interest'. The circumstances should be exceptional and 'in the public interest' is not the same as that which is of interest to the public. In occupational health practice the most likely circumstances are where a worker's health endangers others but the worker refuses the disclosure of information which would allow potential harm to be avoided. Issues may arise in areas such as fitness to drive, communicable diseases or substance abuse in specific groups.   In such circumstances every effort should be made to encourage the worker to consent to disclosure and breach of the duty should only be considered after discussion with senior colleagues and/or a medical defence organisation.

3.82   The Public Interest Disclosure Act 1998 (now the Employment Rights Act 1996) provides that where workers disclose certain types of wrongdoing within, or in limited circumstances outside, their organisation, they are protected from discrimination or dismissal by their employer. In 2012 this legislation is under review. The Act currently applies where a worker has a reasonable belief that:
• a criminal offence has been committed;
• there has been failure to comply with a legal obligation;
• there has been a miscarriage of justice;
• the health and safety of an individual is being endangered;
• the environment is being damaged or;
• there has been deliberate concealment of information tending to show any of the above.

3.83   Occupational health professionals may have information covered by the Act. Before disclosing such information to others (eg the HSE, police and environmental protection agencies) they should consider the issues carefully and consult a legal adviser or their medical defence organisation. It would be very rare to make any disclosure without having discussed matters fully with the company. These ethical duties are likely to override any contractual arrangements including compromise agreements, and the GMC provided specific guidance on this issue in 2012.[53]

VIGNETTE 6 : A problem for the battalion

Captain G was returning from a spell of leave prior to deploying to his operational unit in the Middle East. He had achieved some publicity during his absence due to his having entered a burning house to evacuate trapped persons. At a routine medical assessment abnormal respiratory function tests alerted the medical officer to potential problems. Reduced ventilatory function with a reversible component was considered to be due to smoke inhalation. Major H, the battalion medical officer, advised Captain G that he would have to be listed unfit to deploy and explained in detail that there was a significant risk of exacerbation (especially in a battlefield setting) that would be likely to require intervention and use of scarce medical resources in the field. Captain G declined consent for a medical report indicating his unfitness for deployment to be sent up to Brigade HQ.

Issues

The medical officer has dual duties to both the patient and to those colleagues who would have to rely on Captain G in the field; this could be considered a public interest issue.

Ethical issues relating to unfavourable reports apply equally in both civilian and armed service settings and the hierarchical structure in the armed forces is not a reason for eschewing appropriate ethical behaviour.

Points to consider

How should Major H proceed in this case?

Is it ethically justifiable for him to stand by his decision and report to Brigade HQ that Captain G is unfit to deploy?

4 WORKPLACE HEALTH AND WELLBEING

Introduction

4.1 The scope of occupational health has broadened over time. From simply addressing health issues of the workforce it has extended to take account of the health impact of organisations' products and services, to consider the health of the working age population and to address the impact of work, its inputs and its outputs on society as a whole. In parallel there has been a shift in the paradigm from one which focussed primarily on physical health, to one where mental health is afforded equal importance and beyond, to the concept of wellbeing which incorporates the positive dimension of health in which citizens can realise their potential, work fruitfully and contribute to society.[54]

4.2 The work of occupational health professionals has altered to match this changing landscape. A good understanding of mental health, the management of mental illness and the societal benefits of a positive approach to mental wellbeing are now at least as important as having a firm grasp on the toxicology of chemicals and the effects of physical agents. While the focus on the health of the individual worker remains undiminished, the levers to effect improvements are increasingly recognised as being in the way that work is organised and making an impact on health behaviours in the workplace. As the artificial barriers between occupational health and public health are eroded, the ethical issues faced by occupational health professionals broaden and can become more complex in balancing the needs of the individual with those of wider society.

4.3 Primary prevention of ill-health is a priority for international agencies, national governments and private companies. The drivers are in part the escalating costs of healthcare, but also the realisation that ill-health has a direct impact on productivity through both absenteeism and presenteeism. Early intervention can reduce both the degree and duration of incapacity, making it cost effective for employers to fund such secondary interventions. Tertiary rehabilitation can also reduce employer costs, salvage shortage skills and help to discharge duties related to disability legislation.

Primary prevention

4.4 It is the ethical duty of the occupational health professional to do no harm (non-maleficence) and this is consistent with the risk management hierarchy applied by businesses and the health and safety community. However the occupational health professional also has a duty to do good (beneficence), which does not necessarily translate into traditional management practice though it does accord better with concepts of corporate responsibility. In consequence occupational health professionals may well find themselves acting as advocates for management action for which there is no legal requirement or obvious business requirement and commenting on areas of company activity (eg organisational design) which have not traditionally been viewed as health-related.

Organisational health

4.5 The culture of an organisation and the way that it conducts its activities can have a profound effect upon the health of the workforce. Management style is an important determinant of mental health, and competencies[55] have been developed to help organisations train managers to avoid behaviours which might cause harm and to identify signs of distress in those they manage. Other elements of employment, such as workload, control and change, can affect health, and the perception of justice in the way the organisation behaves is increasingly seen as being critical.[56] Certain working patterns (eg some shift work arrangements) can be harmful to both physical and mental health, while flexibility in working can have both positive and negative effects. Some occupational health professionals still focus only on the narrower issues of hazardous exposures and individual capability, thereby potentially neglecting their wider duty to protect health and promote the wellbeing of people of working age.

4.6 Occupational health professionals need to be aware of these issues and understand the evidence. Only a few will be in a position to influence behaviour directly at an organisational level, but all should flag the issues on an opportunistic basis and link them, where valid, to individual cases on which they are advising. If able to do so, they should then work with colleagues, both clinical and non-clinical, to influence attitudes and behaviours among managers and employee representatives to promote a healthier working environment.

Promotion of health and wellbeing

4.7 The increasing prevalence of non-communicable diseases, including mental health problems, is a global issue.[57] The simple measures of regular exercise, balanced nutrition, tobacco avoidance and alcohol moderation are effective in minimising the risk of disease occurrence and in helping to manage established pathology. Promoting behavioural change in the work environment is particularly effective in public health terms and delivers benefits, not only to the individual worker and society but also to the employing organisation.[58] Occupational health professionals are well placed to promote health and wellbeing in this way, either at the level of the individual worker or by championing workplace schemes.

4.8   Respect for the autonomy of the individual should be paramount when addressing health promotion. Discussions with individuals should set out the evidence in a balanced way that workers are likely to understand and which helps them to make their own decisions. Occupational health professionals should avoid forcing their own views upon others or coercing workers to act in a particular way. They should disassociate themselves from spurious health arguments that others may seek to use in discriminating against workers who engage in habits of which they disapprove. It may be legitimate for employers, in some circumstances, to deny employment to people on the grounds of tobacco use, alcohol consumption, fitness level or physical size. However, occupational health professionals should only engage with this process in so far as those factors have a material impact on the functional capacity of the individual to perform safely the tasks required for the job. Employers should also be made aware that imposing requirements of fitness or physical size or strength unjustifiably may amount to unlawful discrimination on grounds of sex, age or disability.

4.9   When involved in the establishment of health promotion programmes, occupational health professionals should try to ensure that an evidence-based approach is maintained, following published guidelines (eg National Institute for Health and Clinical Excellence)[59-61] where appropriate. The drive to promote wellbeing at work can lead employers to consider offering a range of complementary therapies to their workers. Occupational health professionals should not be dismissive of professionals offering these services but should only endorse those with evidence of effectiveness that meets established scientific standards. A few therapies may be considered actively harmful and occupational health professionals must not only highlight this information to decision makers but also work actively to prevent their introduction. Some therapies may lack scientific proof of benefit but may appear to do no harm and the ethical issue to consider in giving advice is whether providing such services diverts resources from more valuable and proven interventions.

4.10   Participation in health promotion programmes should be voluntary and occupational health professionals should oppose, even well-meaning, compulsion. It is relatively common to offer incentives to workers to encourage their participation but care should be taken to ensure that any disincentives are not punitive. A clear distinction should be drawn between fitness programmes designed to improve operational capability, for example for service personnel and fire-fighters, which may well reasonably be compulsory, and those with more general aspirations to improve health status which should not.

Pre-employment assessment

4.11   The rationale for having any pre-employment health assessment process should be established before it is implemented and the system should be reviewed periodically to ensure that it remains fit for purpose. Criteria to justify such a scheme might include statutory requirements, significant safety risks to the individual, the safety of others, or a material risk to the business by virtue of a critical position held or the associated financial exposure. Few occupations merit the resources required to operate such a system and a number of organisations, including the British Medical Association,[62] recommend a simple enquiry of the selected candidate as to whether they have a health problem or disability for which they might need assistance. Employers rely heavily upon guidance from occupational health professionals when deciding if this service is required and many occupational health professionals rely heavily on this activity to generate income or justify their own positions. Occupational health professionals must be mindful that giving professional advice based on benefit to themselves rather than benefit to their client or the workers they are servicing is unethical, may well be unlawful and could put their healthcare professional registration at risk.

4.12   Having established that there is a requirement for a pre-employment health assessment, the nature of the process must be defined. Asking health questions before an offer of employment has been made is likely to be, or may well be interpreted as being, discriminatory. This has been recognised in equality legislation applicable in Great Britain[63] and it is now unlawful, as a general rule, to make such enquiries until after an offer has been made [see Section 6, Fitness for Work: the legal-ethical interface]. Any assessment should only be undertaken by someone competent to do so; it is self-evident that a health assessment must be carried out by a health professional and, when in relation to employment, that health professional should have suitable and sufficient training in occupational health. Occupational health professionals should disassociate themselves from health assessment processes conducted in whole or in part by administrative staff who are, by definition, not professionally competent for the task. They should seek to change any such systems as being both unethical and ineffective.

4.13   The content of the assessment should reflect the nature of the work to be undertaken. Jobs subject to health surveillance [see paragraph 4.29] should already have content defined and the initial assessment should be consistent with those to be applied during the course of employment. Work that will not be subject to ongoing health surveillance should attract an assessment that takes account of the proposed duties and the risks identified as requiring clearance. There is rarely likely to be any justification for standardised general assessments of health, whether by physical examination or by completion of a health questionnaire. Invading the privacy of individuals by requiring them to disclose sensitive personal information which is not relevant to the assessment process is unethical and may well infringe their human rights. In the UK it also contravenes the principles enshrined in the Data Protection Act[30] which require that information sought is 'adequate, relevant and not excessive in relation to the purpose' and that it is only used for the declared purpose.

4.14　All documentation used to collect pre-employment health data should be suitably marked to show that the information will be held in confidence and usual conditions relating to storage and disclosure apply [see Section 3, Information]. Reports to management should focus on capability and should not include medical detail without the consent of the individual concerned. In general, applicants will be classed as 'fit for the proposed employment' or 'fit subject to defined adjustments'. It is for the prospective employer to determine whether it is reasonable to apply these adjustments and hence whether to confirm the appointment. It is most unusual for an occupational health assessment to result in a decision that an

individual is 'unfit for the proposed employment'. In such cases, it is usually because an applicant has failed to meet predetermined standards. Such standards are often statutory but may be defined on an industry basis or, rarely, in relation to a single organisation. Occupational health professionals involved in setting such standards should ensure that they are, as far as possible, based on capability rather than specific medical conditions and that they are underpinned by robust evidence. Medical standards are inherently discriminatory and those setting and applying them may well have to justify their opinions to an employment tribunal or similar statutory body. Where pre-employment medical standards exist they should be transparent and made available to applicants at an early stage in the recruitment process so that they do not have unrealistic expectations of a job offer.

4.15　A more detailed discussion of the legal principles underpinning pre-employment assessment is presented in Section 6, Fitness for Work: the legal-ethical interface.

Risk control

4.16　Occupational health interventions can play a part in the primary prevention of risk as they relate to both individual workers and to other people. The ethical principles are the same for those in employment as those set out for pre-employment above, even though the legal position may differ.

VIGNETTE 7 : Stringent medical standards exceeding legal requirements

Dr I was a medical officer whose job was to supply occupational health services for several uniformed organisations including security, fire and rescue. Blue light and other response vehicle drivers were expected to undergo health assessment to a standard that was above that required in law. However the standards were considered a requirement of the job. Individuals and trades unions had made representations to occupational health stating that the current medical standards were excessive as they were not a statutory requirement for members of the public undertaking similar roles in industry and commerce. Dr I confirmed this, but explained the safety critical aspects of the roles which often required staff to exceed speed and other limits prescribed in law and, taken together with public perceptions, these required a higher level of fitness. So whilst Dr I agreed that the health requirements were stringent, he did not feel they were excessive in light of the safety critical activities undertaken.

Issues

It is usually difficult to justify setting medical standards outside the statutory framework as they will often be considered discriminatory. The Equality Act permits excluding someone with a disability if it can be justified as a proportionate means of achieving a legitimate aim, which involves a risk assessment and a consideration of possible adjustments.

Individual risk assessment constitutes usual ethical practice, whereby occupational health makes recommendations for adjustments having considered the condition and the employer decides if these are reasonable to implement.

Points to consider

In this example, are the occupational health interventions excessive? Is the risk and public safety argument proportionate to justify the action?

What statutory standards might be considered relevant?

4.17   Where the risk is to the individual, perhaps because of a particular vulnerability to an agent to which they might be exposed in the course of their work, there is a balance to be struck between all four ethical principles [see paragraph 1.13]. In particular, the clinician may have to weigh the autonomy of the worker to decide the acceptability of a risk to their own health or safety against the clinician's duty to do no harm. Medical standards may be helpful in creating a 'yes or no' situation where an individual either meets or fails to meet a defined criterion, but often interpretation is also required.   A paternalistic approach, whereby the clinician makes the decision for the worker, is not acceptable in modern times but neither is an abrogation of responsibility to the individual. Occupational health professionals must explain risks and potential mitigation to the best of their ability and endeavour to do so in language which the worker is likely to understand. The risk should be considered on the basis of the severity of the consequences and the likelihood of occurrence after control measures are taken into account. Occupational health professionals should take time to help the worker come to an informed decision about the level of risk that they find acceptable and then make their own decision on how to act. Every effort should be made to achieve a consensual decision but if the clinician feels that the risk of harm to the individual is too high, regardless of the worker's willingness to accept it, they should follow their conscience and exceptionally refuse to provide medical clearance for the activity. In making such a judgement it would be usual to discuss the issue with experienced colleagues and also to take account of other consequences for the worker, such as loss of income or job security.

4.18   The process for making an ethical decision is similar when the risk of harm includes others apart from the worker.   The worker's autonomy must still be respected, a suitable and sufficient explanation must be given and consensus should be sought. However the balance is shifted toward non-maleficence ('do no harm') and the occupational health professional must weigh the risks to others as well as the risk to the individual worker in arriving at a decision on how to act. In some occupational settings, such as healthcare, the risk to others may be subject to specific provisions[64-68] which may require workers to undergo health surveillance, including testing, as a condition of employment. Occupational health professionals should ensure, as far as they can, that such programmes are rational and evidence-based.

4.19   Where the harm relates to matters other than health and safety, such as legal liability, for which the occupational health professional lacks competence to make a judgement on risk, the consent of the worker should be obtained to pass on appropriate information to the relevant decision maker, such as an employer or insurer. The normal provisions regarding the disclosure of personal information will apply [see paragraphs 3.59-3.62].   If the worker does not consent to pass on information in this way then the clinician may deem the assessment process to have been frustrated and may refuse to provide medical clearance for the activity.

Immunisation

4.20   Immunisation against occupational biohazards is another aspect of hazard control. The ethical issues again are influenced by whether the programme is primarily for the protection of the individual worker (where autonomy is likely to be most important) or for the protection of others (where non-maleficence becomes critical). This purpose must be clearly defined from the outset and should be explicit in all instructions to occupational health professionals and to workers; involving workers' representatives in the design and communication of programmes can be helpful.   An ethical complication of immunisation, unlike most health assessments, is that the procedure itself may cause harm to the individual worker and it may not always convey the desired protection; any programme must be planned taking these factors into account. Immunisation is also invasive and failure to obtain consent is therefore not just unethical but, potentially, an assault. Occupational health professionals should ensure that policies are clear about how workers who fail to develop the anticipated immunity following vaccination will be managed and that individuals have been apprised of this information before entering the programme. Similarly the approach to dealing with workers who decline immunisation should be determined and promulgated in advance of implementing a programme.

4.21   Some immunisations,   notably against influenza, are offered partly for the protection of workers and those with whom they come into contact (including, in the National Health Service (NHS), potentially vulnerable patients) but have the additional benefit for organisations of trying to mitigate the operational disruption of sickness absence. Occupational health professionals should understand the reasons behind such programmes and must not misrepresent the benefits to workers. This extension of the beneficence argument beyond the individual being immunised is plausible but tenuous and occupational health professionals should reflect on its validity in their own situation.

International assignments

4.22   A number of organisations require staff to operate for extended periods in parts of the world remote from their homeland. Such postings, in which the worker may be accompanied by their family, can be to areas where health risks are greater than in their home geography or local healthcare facilities are more basic. Occupational health professionals may be asked to advise on the suitability of workers and their families for such assignments. Factors to consider include:

- does the worker or family member have a condition which would be exacerbated by factors in the proposed environment?
- is the worker or family member particularly vulnerable to diseases endemic in the proposed environment?
- is the worker or family member likely to require a level of healthcare not readily available in the proposed environment?
- is the worker likely to experience a period of extended incapacity during the assignment?
- is the worker likely to require evacuation out of the area or region for treatment?

4.23   The ethical considerations are the same as for those outlined in the hazard control section [see paragraphs 4.17-4.19], namely balancing the principles of autonomy and non-maleficence. Occupational health professionals should be mindful that international assignments are often lucrative for individuals and may enhance career progression – workers may therefore be tempted to take a higher degree of risk in relation to health issues. Conversely, the nature of such assignments is often 'mission critical' and the organisation may have a low appetite for risk. Occupational health professionals are rarely the decision makers in such cases and quantifying risks on a sound evidence base and presenting the issues cogently to all concerned is therefore essential.

Secondary intervention

4.24   Early intervention in the context of occupational health may relate to the individual worker, a working population or the employing organisation. Taking action in this way must be justified by an anticipated generation of benefits which outweigh the costs incurred. Both costs and benefits have multiple dimensions and occupational health professionals must evaluate their actions in more than simple financial terms, taking account of the ethical requirements for both beneficence and non-maleficence. Consideration must also be given to where the costs and benefits accrue. The traditional medical model in its simplest form sees both elements affecting solely the patient (worker) but that is rarely the case in modern practice. It is now much more common for costs to be borne by a third party, either on a shared risk basis through insurance or taxation or, as is normal in the world of employment, as a cost of doing business. Ethical questions can therefore arise about what is a reasonable threshold at which to cap organisational costs for a given benefit to an individual.

4.25   Perhaps more difficult is the situation where the action is taken to benefit parties other than the individual worker. The beneficiary may be the funding organisation, other workers or the general public, but the cost to the individual worker may be substantial in loss of earnings or even employment. Ethical analysis

---

VIGNETTE 8 : Complexities of an overseas assignment

Dr J was employed by a government agency as medical team leader to assess individuals and their families prior to postings abroad. During a routine nurse-led assessment it became apparent that there were complex issues concerning the proposed posting of Mr K to a remote and malaria prone area of sub-Saharan Africa. This was an accompanied post; Mr K's wife was nineteen weeks pregnant (and her first pregnancy had ended in miscarriage at six months); one of the two teenage sons also accompanying had special educational needs, Asperger's Syndrome and ADHD. It was clear that due to the nature and rural location of the post it would be unsuitable for both the employee's son and also his wife as there would be a complete lack of appropriate resources and support.

Issues

There are competing ethical considerations here, including the autonomy of the individuals concerned to make personal decisions about level of risk balanced against the company liability for the health and safety of its workers.

There is no duty to make adjustments, reasonable or unreasonable, for the parent of a disabled child. Under the Equality Act 2010 only direct discrimination and discriminatory harassment are covered by associative discrimination.

In these circumstances, occupational health professionals have a duty to identify potential risks to the employer (which may include high costs and operational disruption), as well as potential issues for the individuals (limitations of healthcare and educational resources in many locations).

Points to consider

What possible solutions are there in this situation? Is cancellation the only option?

Is it ethical to collude with pressure from workers and their employers to 'make things work'?

---

therefore needs to be wider than simply balancing benefit and harm and must consider the autonomy of the individual as well as the justice of the action taken and its likely consequences.

Health screening

4.26 Well person health screening is defined by the UK National Screening Committee as:

'a process of identifying apparently healthy people who may be at increased risk of a disease or condition. They can then be offered information, further tests and appropriate treatment to reduce their risk and/or any complications arising from the disease or condition.'[69]

4.27 Screening may be offered by employers as part of a remuneration package, to help moderate health insurance costs or to complement other health promotion activities. However, once taken up, it is an activity for the sole benefit of the individual worker. It must be differentiated from health surveillance which is an activity undertaken as part of a hazard control programme or to ensure continuing fitness to work where there are specific health criteria. Health screening programmes should be evidence-based and, to be ethically acceptable, should satisfy established criteria such as those published by the UK National Screening Committee.[70] Those criteria are a development of the ones developed by Wilson and Jungner[71] in 1968 and may be summarised as:

- all primary prevention should have been implemented as far as is reasonably practicable;
- tests must be safe, simple, acceptable and validated;
- testing should be directed at an important health

problem;
- the condition should be understood;
- further investigation and, where necessary, treatment should be readily available;
- strong evidence that screening reduces mortality or morbidity should be available.

Adhering to a framework such as this is valuable in dealing with the commercial conflict of interest that occupational health professionals can face with some screening where benefits are marginal or poorly demonstrated.

4.28 Screening is a voluntary activity and while occupational health professionals may encourage and promote participation, they must avoid being complicit in programmes that use compulsion. Where screening is conducted by an occupational health professional, or by staff for whom they have professional responsibility, they must ensure that facilities, equipment and training are all suitable and sufficient for the task being undertaken. If screening is outsourced, the occupational health professional should ensure that the chosen organisation operates to valid protocols and in accordance with recognised standards, where appropriate. Arrangements must be in place for the follow-up of abnormal results, including referral with consent to the worker's own medical professionals. Aggregated results of workforce screening may be used to demonstrate the impact of programmes or to provide a picture of the health of the workforce provided the response to screening is sufficient to ensure the validity of the data. It is

---

VIGNETTE 9 : Health screening – occupational health involvement in non-statutory monitoring

Dr L had recently been appointed head of occupational health in an organisation employing several thousand workers. He discovered that the occupational health department was offering annual cervical cytology screening for all women (average age 36) requesting it. This programme had been started after the death of an employee from cervical cancer. Another programme offered workers capillary blood cholesterol screening. At the same time as occupational health nurses were carrying out this non-statutory activity unrelated to work, they were also under pressure to attend to routine risk-related health assessments in employees undertaking a wide range of hazardous activities in their work.

Issues

While it is not unethical for employers to offer workers health-related activities beyond statutory requirements, when occupational health resource is limited consideration must be given to activities that give best value for money in maximising worker health, wellbeing and safety.

Where screening is available as part of a quality assured national screening programme it would be unethical for employers to offer interventions that did not meet all the standards of an effective and evidence-based screening programme.

Points to consider

What should Dr L do in this situation? Who should be involved in any decisions to change established practice?

If the cervical cytology screening programme were to be terminated, how should this be explained to the workforce?

Is executive screening ethical?

---

essential that data used in this way are anonymised and presented in a way that prevents linkage to identifiable individuals.

Health surveillance

4.29   It is important to distinguish between health screening, which is primarily for the benefit of the worker, and health surveillance which is part of a hazard control programme. While the former is voluntary the latter is not and is usually a condition of employment in a given role. The aim of health surveillance, in the context of secondary intervention, is to identify physiological changes that might indicate the early signs of toxicity or changes in health status that might increase a worker's vulnerability. The ethical issues in ongoing health surveillance include those that need to be considered in primary prevention, but the impact on the worker of the occupational health professional's decision is usually greater. Denying someone an opportunity to work is a major decision but taking their livelihood away is even more significant. Decisions must be based on sound evidence which should be confirmed if there is material doubt. Professional judgement must be objective and must not be swayed unduly by emotion, but compassion should be shown in communicating adverse results to the worker. Matters requiring medical intervention should be referred appropriately and agreement should be sought from the worker to communicate the employment outcome (but not the health issues) to the employer. If the worker refuses consent for the outcome to be communicated, the occupational health professional must consider whether a public interest disclosure is indicated or whether it will suffice to advise the employer that health surveillance could not be completed because of withdrawal of consent.

Biological monitoring

4.30   Programmes for biological monitoring and biological effect monitoring must have a clear purpose and be well planned and implemented. The outcome should be improved control of hazards and reduction of risk. Participation should include consent even when monitoring is required by law. Although the purpose of the programme may be to use the grouped results to assess and improve control measures, individual results falling outside agreed parameters will require specialist interpretation. Arrangements should be in place to refer, if considered necessary.

4.31   Planning such programmes must include the communication of results. The release of grouped results to all those with an interest in the control of the risks must be agreed in advance. Occasionally it may be necessary to release an individual's results to a third party to achieve the objective, but this can only be with their consent.

Drug and alcohol testing

4.32   Testing programmes operate at the boundaries between a worker's private life and their employment. Programmes should therefore only be introduced after careful consideration of the full implications for the way an organisation wishes to engage with its workforce, and early consultation between social partners is prudent. Clarity of purpose for any drug and alcohol testing programmes is essential and these should only be introduced in general for safety critical tasks. Care should be taken that health and safety is not used as an excuse to introduce measures underpinned by other motives such as enhancing corporate image, and proportionality is an important principle to apply. In general, alcohol is easier to deal with because consumption is lawful in most jurisdictions and the pharmaco-kinetics are relatively predictable. The illegal nature of many recreational drugs, the potential for confusion with prescribed medication, the lack of easily demonstrable dose-effect relationships, and the persistence of some substances create practical problems as well as potential civil liberties and human rights issues that must be considered. No programme should be introduced without a detailed policy that sets out the reasons for testing, the procedures to be followed and any role for occupational health professionals. Consideration should be given to how unintended consequences, such as the detection of disease markers, will be managed. Many organisations employ specialist contractors to conduct testing programmes since this avoids potential conflict of interest for occupational health professionals and removes potential confusion among workers about the role of the service. This issue is the subject of detailed guidance produced by the Faculty of Occupational Medicine[72] and others.[73]

Genetic testing and monitoring

4.33   Neither genetic testing nor monitoring is yet well developed but knowledge is increasing rapidly and tests are becoming more widely available. Providers of testing facilities are likely to seek to grow their market and employment is a logical area in which they may seek to expand. Genetic tests may be undertaken in a number of circumstances, predominantly outside the work context. Examples of different test types are set out in the table overleaf:

4.34   Employers might feel that they want genetic information about their workers for a number of reasons including:
- to protect the public where employees with a genetic condition could represent a serious danger to others;
- to identify a worker's susceptibility to the effects of particular toxic or carcinogenic agents in an occupational environment;
- to detect damage caused by a workplace exposure

Test Type	Description
Screening	Population testing without cause for increased risk of future disease (eg dementia)
Diagnostic	Confirmation of suspected disease with a view to improved condition management (eg familial bowel cancer)
Pre-symptomatic	Testing of asymptomatic people at known risk to provide information on chances of developing future disease (eg Huntington's chorea)
Carrier status	Testing to identify potential risks of the next generation developing disease (eg cystic fibrosis)
Susceptibility	Testing for increased susceptibility to toxic agents (eg beryllium) or physical risks (eg carpal tunnel syndrome)
Monitoring	Use of DNA damage to identify early toxic effects of an agent before signs of disease (eg carcinogens)

to an agent in advance of physiological effects or disease;

- to assess a job applicant's long-term health prospects.

4.35   Carrier status is only likely to be of interest to an employer if medical insurance is provided for family members. In the UK testing for health insurance purposes is ruled out, with minor exceptions, by a moratorium agreed between the insurance industry and the Government; the long standing agreement was extended in 2011 until 2017. In the USA, where health insurance is a more prominent feature of employment, testing for these purposes is prohibited by the Genetic Information Non-discrimination Act (2008).

4.36   There are isolated instances of testing being used to discriminate against job applicants. This may well run counter to Article 6 of the Universal Declaration of the Human Genome and Human Rights. More information is available from the Human Genetics Commission and the Emerging Science and Bioethics Advisory Committee which replaced the Commission in 2012.[74] A genetic defect is not a disability under the Equality Act until it becomes symptomatic.

4.37   Criteria for voluntary genetic testing in the workplace[75] have been developed and may be helpful in advising employers in this complex area. All six requirements must be met:

- A genetic test (for a specific condition) must be available which is highly *specific and sensitive* and offers an acceptably low incidence of both false positives and false negatives; such a test must test for a gene that is sufficiently penetrant for the test result to have some important health implication.
- Testing should be carried out by an independent laboratory, and *results of genetic tests* should be given to workers directly, either by a geneticist or a genetic counsellor; test results should be held in confidence, and revealed to the employer only at the employee's request.

- Pre- and post-test genetic *counselling* must be available from a qualified health professional, and paid for by the employer, regardless of the outcome of the test.
- The gene being tested for must not be prominently associated with an identifiable and historically *disadvantaged group*.
- Where relevant, the employer must guarantee continued access to *group insurance*.
- The employer must ensure that if the employee chooses to reveal that she has tested positive, suitable policies are in place to ensure a reasonable degree of *job security*.

Tertiary rehabilitation

4.38   Helping the sick or injured to recover capability and return to productive employment is at the heart of occupational health. Integrating knowledge of health issues, work activity and the workplace environment allows advice to be given that can benefit both the worker and the employer. In some circumstances occupational health professionals advise on the provision of, or act as the gateway to, specific services geared to promoting effective rehabilitation and ethical issues are akin to those discussed in relation to early intervention. More often difficulties arise when one or other party in the employment relationship is driven by motives which compromise a smooth return to work and occupational health professionals can come under pressure to slant their advice. This can be compounded where occupational health professionals have duties to third parties, such as regulatory authorities or pension schemes, or where their opinion on capability differs from that of the worker's own medical advisers.

4.39   A more detailed discussion of the law underpinning fitness for work considerations is set out in Section 6, Fitness for Work: the legal-ethical interface.

Supporting sick workers

4.40   Occupational health professionals may have

the opportunity to engage with sick workers while they are still working normally and the aim should be to give them, and their employer, advice which will help them to continue working safely and as effectively as possible while accessing suitable and sufficient treatment. However, sick workers are often only referred for occupational health input once they have commenced a spell of sickness absence. Such referrals may be part of an absence management process and occupational health professionals should ensure that their prime focus remains the welfare of the individual worker, and not the absence or its impact on the organisation. There is an emphasis in modern occupational health practice on the report of a consultation but occupational health professionals must neither neglect the advice they can give to the sick worker, nor underestimate the impact that they can have in influencing the health and wellbeing of the person they are seeing. Workers must be treated with courtesy and respect, recognising that an occupational health assessment may well be a new experience for many which they could find threatening or intimidating. Assessments should be as comprehensive as the circumstances dictate and opinions formulated should be objective and non-judgemental. Care should be taken not to undermine the worker's confidence in the treatment they are receiving from their own professionals, but any clinical concerns should be explored and followed up. Information which might be of benefit in improving the worker's treatment should, with consent, be passed on to the treating professional; this is normally best effected in writing but, if that is not practicable, oral instructions to the worker should be recorded in the occupational health records.

Recommending adjustments

4.41   Temporary adjustments can be an important element in helping workers make a successful transition from sickness absence to work. Occupational health professionals should use their training and experience to help define adjustments that will make a difference and there is a growing evidence base upon which they can rely. However, adjustments can only help if they are implemented, and occupational health professionals have a duty to ensure that what they recommend is likely to make sense and be acceptable to the worker and the employer. It is for the employer to determine whether it is reasonable to make a specific adjustment, but the occupational health professional who recommends totally unrealistic measures, even with a theoretical basis, is behaving irresponsibly and unethically.

4.42   Permanent adjustments and alternative duties are usually more difficult to accommodate in the workplace than temporary measures. Occupational health professionals should give very careful consideration before issuing advice that may render an individual unemployable. Many workers have an incorrect and naïve view of the power of occupational health professionals and think that guidance they give must be followed by employers. They may therefore welcome occupational health statements which they perceive as making their working lives easier without realising the longer term implications. Occupational health professionals may gain temporary satisfaction or avoid interpersonal conflict by telling workers what they think they want to hear, but that is not responsible behaviour. Recommendations that offer a desirable benefit to the worker at the expense of costing them their job do not represent sound ethical judgement.

Conflicting advice

4.43   Workers may report that the employment advice they have received from their treating healthcare professionals is at odds with the opinion of the occupational health professional. Less commonly, treating healthcare professionals indicate that they have given such advice. There is rarely value in engaging in confrontation on this issue since that is unlikely to result in resolution and the worker will have their trust undermined in their own clinicians, occupational health or both. It is unprofessional to denigrate the views of other clinicians and occupational health professionals may find that taking the stated position as a starting point from which to negotiate movement to their own opinion over time is a productive approach. In the absence of material movement it may be necessary to state simply that views differ and close the discussion; it should be understood that workers will generally favour the opinions of their treating professionals and/or those which they perceive to be most beneficial. Employers are entitled to prefer the opinion of their professional occupational health advisers [see Section 6, Fitness for Work: the legal-ethical interface].

Termination of employment

4.44   Occupational health professionals rarely have direct involvement in the termination of workers' employment but they do often provide information critical to the process. In attendance cases input usually centres on prognosis, either in relation to a single extended absence or with regard to the impact of an underlying condition on repeated absences. Occupational health professionals have a duty to provide realistic estimates based on sound evidence – undue optimism or pessimism is inappropriate and can cause harm to the worker and/or the employer. Poor performance may have a health component and, again, a realistic estimate of the contribution made by ill-health and the future outlook are required. In discipline cases health status may constitute either a defence or mitigation for sentence. In both cases it is essential to obtain accurate evidence and to link it to the time of the alleged offence. Impaired mental health is common in discipline cases but it often relates to the process and potential penalty rather than being a pre-existing

---

VIGNETTE 10 : Different opinions

Mr M had worked for the past fifteen years for a major investment bank. He was taken ill at work and, in Accident & Emergency, was diagnosed with a myocardial infarction and he was referred urgently for angioplasty. He had not previously suffered any cardiac symptoms but he smoked 10 cigarettes a day, was moderately overweight and had recognised for a while that he should be doing something to reduce the stress he experienced in a normal working day. On discharge from hospital Mr M had been signed off sick for six weeks but towards the end of this period he brought his manager a GP 'fit note' that signed him off sick for a further three months and recommended a return to half-time hours for four months subsequent to this.

The company's in-house occupational health doctor, Dr N, considered Mr M ready for rehabilitation from six weeks following his discharge from hospital and Mr M's manager identified a number of short-term projects that took Mr M away from the pressures of his usual role. However Mr M told his manager that he would not be returning to work until his GP was happy for him to do so.

Issues

Conflicts of advice may arise in situations where there is an incomplete understanding of the situation, for example possibilities for adaptations to work requirements. Different parties may have conflicting motives, or mistaken beliefs around what is helpful in a given situation.

Employers and workers do seek alternative opinions. The issue for occupational health is to encourage dialogue wherever possible to achieve satisfactory resolution to the differences.

Points to consider

What can occupational health do to help Mr M comfortably achieve an earlier return to work?

How should Dr N handle the conflict of advice between himself and the GP?

---

condition that might have influenced the conduct in question.

4.45   It is not unusual for workers faced with performance and discipline cases to take extended certificated sick leave. Occupational health professionals may well be asked to determine whether a worker is fit to attend investigation and resolution meetings. The key issues are whether the worker is capable of understanding the case against him and of replying to the charges, either in person or by instructing a representative. It may well be the case that the worker will find the proceedings distressing but that delaying the process for a prolonged period is likely to be more damaging to his health. This is an issue poorly understood by many workers, their representatives and their own healthcare professionals. The occupational health professional should try to explain to all concerned the concept of doing least harm, and guidance can usefully be supplemented by advice on the provision of support, choice of meeting venue, etc. Employers may choose to conduct proceedings in the absence of the worker if refusal to attend becomes protracted, but this is rarely in the best interests of the worker and should only be done after several attempts have been made to engage with the worker, either in person or through representatives.

Health-related pension benefits

4.46   The virtual demise of defined benefit pension schemes in the private sector, in favour of defined contribution schemes, has greatly reduced the need for occupational health advice in this area. Nevertheless, defined benefit schemes continue for the time being in much of the public sector and occupational health input is often sought in relation to enhanced benefits payable for medical retirement and in some cases for injury awards. Ethical responsibilities in this area are more complex than in much of occupational health because stakeholders include the pension scheme administrators and trustees as well as the workers and the employers. Occupational health professionals must be particularly clear about where their responsibilities lie, both in their own minds and in the way that they communicate with others. In many schemes there is now a separation of functions between occupational health employment guidance and the provision of advice to the pension authorities. Occupational health professionals must take care not to offer gratuitous advice on eligibility for benefits when it is not their responsibility to do so, since that may raise false expectations and thereby cause harm.

4.47   Occupational health professionals advising pension schemes must fully understand the eligibility criteria and their interpretation. Many schemes have similar criteria but the transposition of words and phrases can alter meaning significantly, for example 'permanent incapacity due to ill-health' is a more stringent requirement than 'incapacity due to permanent ill-health'. If the criteria include reference to the worker's job, as is common, the occupational health professional should have suitable and sufficient knowledge of what that work entails so that a valid

VIGNETTE 11 : Considering eligibility for ill-health retirement and early release of benefits

Dr O had recently been appointed as pension scheme advisor for a large insurance group. For her first case the trustees had referred the case of Mr P, a 61-year-old middle manager in a soft drinks manufacturing company. He had been off sick for more than a year following an episode of chest pain whilst cycling home from work. Immediate intervention and the insertion of a coronary artery stent had produced excellent medical results with no cardiac sequelae; however he had not returned to work. He had now exhausted his employer's sickness benefits and was in receipt of state benefits. Senior management had attempted unsuccessfully to encourage rehabilitation and a phased return to work and their frustration had now resulted in a referral to the company pension scheme for consideration of ill-health retirement, ie early release of benefits.

Dr O had to hand three encouraging and optimistic hospital reports and two GP reports, which hinted at a degree of reluctance in the employee to return to work. Although she could have based her advice on the reports alone, Dr O considered that she needed to see and examine the employee. She found little to convince herself of any permanent incapacity. Mr P requested a sight of the report and immediately questioned the relevance of a comment that he was now settled in his holiday home on the coast of mainland Europe. Dr O agreed to remove that remark from her report, which was then sent to the trustees with Mr P's consent. The trustees rejected the application and the scheme administrator wrote to Mr P to explain that he would not be entitled to pension benefits until the age of 65.

Issues

Consent needs to be sought if there is new disclosure, for example as a result of the consultation and examination. For information that has already been disclosed, a report can be released without the need to seek consent from the individual concerned. However the individual is entitled to be sent a copy of the report under the Data Protection Act.

When making decisions on ill-health retirement applications, occupational health professionals must have a clear understanding of the rules applicable to each individual pension scheme and reflect on best evidence for good medical practice to consider prognosis.

Points to consider

Would it have been ethical for Dr O to issue a report to the trustees without having seen Mr P first? Would that alter the consent procedures?

judgement can be made. Assessments may be made on the basis of a physical consultation or as a 'papers only' process. Neither is inherently superior from an ethical standpoint – a physical consultation may convey the perception of greater autonomy for the worker but it also runs a greater risk of partiality arising from an emotional response to the applicant's situation. The foremost responsibility in these cases is to the pension scheme and, of the four ethical principles, justice is therefore predominant.

5   OCCUPATIONAL HEALTH RESEARCH

Introduction

5.1   Research is essential to the successful development of evidence-based practice in occupational health and a healthy research sector is vital to the continuing protection of people at work. Many occupational health professionals will engage in research during training and for some this is a required part of accreditation. The need to undertake research may also arise as part of professional practice, for example investigating a disease cluster or emerging occupational risk factors. There is increasing regulation and heightened societal expectation that research will respect the rights and privacy of the individual, even if there is potential for public benefit. Therefore the careful management of ethical problems is an important and integral component of good research practice. Most funded research in occupational health is carried out through academic centres that should have established procedures and access to expertise in this area, but all occupational health professionals should have an understanding of the main ethical issues that might arise.

Determining what constitutes research

5.2   A common area of difficulty for occupational health professionals is deciding whether the activity they wish to undertake constitutes research or not. Research has been defined in the following way:

Research aims to generate (new) information, knowledge, understanding, or some other relevant cognitive good, and does so by means of a systematic investigation.[76]

5.3   The definition and classifications of research are, however, not always clear.[77] The distinction between research, audit (designed to inform delivery of best care through assessment against a 'gold' standard) and service development/evaluation (designed to define or judge current care) is important to clarify [see table at end of this section]. In practice these categories may not be mutually exclusive. Guidance from the United Bristol Healthcare NHS Trust[78] specifically discusses 'grey areas' noting for the 'researcher' that 'you may still find yourself struggling to decide whether your proposed project is audit or research. Indeed it is possible that larger projects may contain elements of both audit and research...'. For the occupational health professional the investigation of a disease cluster, health surveillance and biological monitoring programmes may be added to the list of activities which may be considered to fall into this 'grey area'.

Independent ethical review

5.4   For the purposes of determining whether an activity is ethical these distinctions matter little because the principles and their interpretation in the context of occupational health practice are the same. Good practice is ethical practice and 'decisions about the need for ethical review should be based on the morality of all actions rather than arbitrary distinctions between audit and research'.[79] The distinction becomes important, however, in defining the need for an independent ethical review of the work, generally by a research ethics committee, and here there are two determining factors:

- There is a specific statutory requirement for independent ethical review. One example in occupational health practice from the UK would be obtaining biological samples which are considered 'relevant tissue' under the Human Tissue Act 2004. If these are obtained during the course of the research (a scheduled process under the Act) then independent ethical review by a recognised research ethics committee is a statutory requirement unless the samples can be held/stored in a facility licensed by the Human Tissue Authority. If the tissue is obtained for the purposes of audit, quality control or statutory health surveillance it is not subject to these requirements. Another example is the tracing of subjects in occupational cohort studies through the NHS Information Centre.

- The governance arrangements of the controlling organisation require independent ethical review. The majority of universities and the UK NHS require independent ethical review for research, but not for audit and service evaluation. The rationale is based on a broad consideration of 'risk' to the health and wellbeing of those participating in the 'study'. Research, with little or no benefit to the participant, is perceived as being relatively high risk and therefore subject to significant ethical concerns, whilst audit and service evaluation, having potential benefit for participants, are considered relatively low risk with 'no significant material ethical issues'.

5.5   Strict interpretation of these factors might lead to the conclusion that all research involving human volunteers, their tissue or personal data, has the potential for raising ethical concerns and therefore should be submitted to independent ethical review. However, such independent reviews are onerous and the principle of proportionality should be applied to avoid placing an unnecessary burden on both the research process and the ethical review mechanism.

The principle requires the level of ethical review to be proportionate to the risks faced by volunteers from their participation in the research and is addressed more fully subsequently in paragraphs 5.30-5.31.

Ethical research and research guidelines

5.6   It is important that researchers together with any 'sponsor(s)' (ie the individual, or organisation (or group of individuals or organisations) that takes on responsibility for confirming there are proper arrangements to initiate, manage, monitor, and finance a study) consider ethical issues from the early stages of a research project. From the beginning of the design process, provisional decisions are usually taken about the nature of the research sample and of the methodology. Inevitably these decisions imply certain ways of interacting with the people involved in the research. Investigators must therefore be skilled not only in the scientific aspects of research, but also have the training to be aware of and implement appropriate ethical standards.

5.7   Research activity is defined in terms of general aims and specific objectives which will often highlight potential ethical issues, because they imply certain forms of methodology and of data collection. For example, the aim of research may be to explore individual differences within relatively small numbers of subjects; any participants must understand the purpose and function of such research before agreeing to take part. Conversely research aims might involve making large-scale comparisons between groups of subjects; data can be combined to obscure identity and obviate disclosure issues. It is therefore essential to consider ethical issues from the outset in relation to all programmes. This is a precursor to deciding whether reference to a research ethics committee is warranted; independent review is not a substitute for reflective analysis.

Guidelines

5.8   The first reference to ethical issues and research (experimental medicine) is that of Thomas Percival's code from 1803 which specified that 'the physician may try experimental treatments when all else fails, and when it can serve the public good'.[80] The norms of contemporary research ethics were codified by the Nuremberg Code of 1947 in response to Nazi medical research and this has been further developed by the World Medical Association.[81] The principles set out in the introduction to this Faculty guidance underpin research ethics as well as other areas of practice.

5.9   Drawing on these principles, Emanuel and colleagues have defined seven requirements that provide a systematic and coherent framework for determining whether clinical research is ethical.[82] These are summarised by the authors and in the current context can be restated as being:

- **Social or scientific value:** evaluation of a treatment, intervention, or theory that has potential to improve health and wellbeing or increase knowledge.
- **Scientific validity**: use of widely acceptable scientific principles and methods, including statistical techniques, to produce reliable and valid data.
- **Fair subject selection**: selection of participants so that vulnerable individuals are not unfairly targeted for risky research and the rich and socially powerful not favoured for potentially beneficial research.
- **Favourable risk-benefit ratio**: minimization of risks; enhancement of potential benefits; risks to the participant are proportionate to the benefits to the participant, the workforce as a whole and society.
- **Independent review**: where appropriate review the research protocol, its proposed participant population, and risk-benefit ratio by individuals unaffiliated with the research.
- **Consent**: provision of information to participants about purpose of the research, its procedures, potential risks, benefits, and alternatives, so that the individual understands this information and can make a voluntary decision whether to enrol and continue to participate.
- **Respect for potential and enrolled subjects**: respect for participants by:
  - o   permitting withdrawal from the research;
  - o   protecting privacy through confidentiality;
  - o   informing participants of newly discovered risks or benefits;
  - o   providing participants the opportunity to receive the results of the research;
  - o   maintaining welfare of participants.

5.10   Most occupational health research projects are conducted outside a therapeutic setting and involve approaches to individual members of a workforce or healthy volunteers. Although some interventional studies are conducted by occupational health professionals, most research involves observational methods (eg cohort or case-control designs) examining workers' performance of their normal day-to-day work activities. Alternatively, studies may be population based involving the analysis of existing health or database records. The ethical issues may therefore differ from clinical research and reference to guidance specific to occupational health research practice, such as that produced by Rothstein,[83] may be helpful. Research for professional accreditation or requiring independent review by a research ethics committee should normally involve formal affiliation with an academic unit or the NHS.

5.11 Most occupational health research would fall into the 'low risk' category of clinical research. The ethical issues tend to centre on recruitment, consent, confidentiality, data protection and communication.

Information governance in research

Consent

5.12 Those recruited to an occupational health research study as active participants must give free and informed consent as with other occupational health activities [see paragraphs 3.37-3.38]. An example of where it may not be practical to obtain consent is from ex-employees for participation in a retrospective cohort study of mortality and cancer incidence. Issues can arise in a workplace setting in relation to whether participation is truly 'voluntary'. Coercion must not be used and clarification of the relationship between the study team and the employer is often important in this regard. Due attention should be paid to the perception of workers and whether the presentation of the research might make them feel that their employment position could be affected, adversely or favourably, by their decision on whether to participate. Similarly, misrepresentation of the societal importance of the research or the possible impact on workers' personal health status is unethical. Information for workers about the purpose, risks and benefits of the research should be presented in a way and in language that they are likely to understand. The level of detail should be neither too complex nor too vague and be pitched at what a reasonable person would need to know, or want to know, in order to decide whether to participate. Workers participating in research should be regarded as a vulnerable group, because of the power relationship that exists with the employer, and they should be afforded additional protection beyond that normally provided to research participants.[84] Involving workers' representatives at an early stage in study development can be helpful in avoiding some of these pitfalls.

5.13 Specific issues that should be addressed include:
- the identity of the research team (for example in-house occupational health providers, or an independent academic team);
- arrangements for access to counselling or other sources of advice to mitigate any identified potential harm or distress;
- a complaints procedure and arrangements for compensation in the event of study related injury;
- data usage and safeguards, including information on how the study will be reported;
- a participant information sheet;[85]
- an oral presentation or briefing;
- sources of further information;
- a defined time, at least 24 hours, to make a decision before giving any consent (although participants in postal questionnaire studies will make their own decision if wishing to reply sooner);
- express consent as the norm, with full justification where implied consent is relied upon (see below);
- provide the opportunity for targeted feedback to subjects.

5.14 An example where it might be justified to imply consent is that of the questionnaire survey – the act of completing the questionnaire implies consent. However, implied consent still needs to be informed and relevant information should be provided either in an accompanying letter or information sheet, or it should be included as a preamble to the questionnaire itself. It should not be assumed, however, that all questionnaire surveys are minimal or 'low risk' (even if anonymous) and hence implied consent and cursory ethical review justified. Questionnaires may involve reference to sensitive issues (those likely to cause embarrassment or lead to discrimination, for example HIV status) and these will need to be highlighted and presented in the information to (potential) participants. Such questionnaire research might also be expected to have undergone independent ethical review. Researchers must also be aware of intrusive questioning, for example a research questionnaire unnecessarily requesting a construction worker to provide his National Insurance number may be considered an invasion of privacy.

5.15 Care must be taken not to confuse research with health surveillance and it is improper to 'pass off' one as the other. Occupational health professionals must remember that consent only applies to the activity and the purpose for which it was sought. Where a dataset is compiled for one purpose, with express consent, but is then proposed for analysis in unrelated research with different objectives, consideration must be given to the need for further consent. This will apply whether the original data was obtained in a research context or during routine occupational health practice.

Confidentiality and data protection

5.16 The normal occupational health arrangements relating to confidentiality and data protection apply to research [see paragraphs 3.5-3.9]. As with the provision of management information, research information should be anonymised (stripped of any information that might enable identification of the individual) at the earliest opportunity. It should be noted that linked anonymised (pseudonymised) or coded data do not constitute properly anonymised data. Data that is already anonymised at the point of access will not normally fall within the scope of data protection legislation. If it is proposed that routine occupational health records or personal exposure data might be used to generate anonymised information for research purposes, the occupational health professional must, where possible, ensure that employees are informed prospectively. Workers should be told that their data might be used for research, how it might be used and how confidentiality will be protected. It is prudent to consult with worker representatives at an early stage in the process.

5.17   If subsequent access to occupational health records is requested by a third party (such as an academic team) for research purposes, the occupational health professional must ensure that the third party has appropriate procedures to comply with the principles of data protection, and that all personnel accept a duty of confidence. Wherever possible, workers' consent for disclosure of personal identifiable information should be sought: however, if the data is anonymised to the researcher this additional consent is not necessary. Particular care should be taken with smaller groups of workers where anonymised data may still allow for identification of an individual. In all cases the minimum information necessary should be disclosed.

5.18   Specific provisions apply to some organisations, such as the UK NHS, where the use of patient information for research purposes without consent in the public interest is allowed by law, subject to defined safeguards.[86] These provisions have enabled the lawful use of patient information in special circumstances, for example by cancer registries, which would otherwise be at risk of failure to comply with the duty of confidence. Whether the use of data without consent is justifiable in a particular study can be difficult to judge. Medical Research Council (MRC) guidance outlines the aspects that must be taken into account, including the necessity and importance of the research, the sensitivity of the information used, the steps taken to safeguard personal data, and the opinion of an independent research ethics committee.[87] Neither compliance with published guidance nor ethics committee approval guarantees that actions are ethical, or even that they will withstand legal challenge. Occupational health professionals who access personal information for research purposes must therefore undertake their own ethical analysis, take account of the statutory framework and be prepared to justify their actions.

5.19   The recruitment process to a study can, of itself, compromise confidentiality. If inclusion criteria require having a particular health condition then, by virtue of volunteering, workers risk this personal information becoming 'public' knowledge. Similarly screening out people who do not meet specific criteria from a recruited population runs the risk that sensitive information may be inferred. Calling/recruitment notices should therefore focus on exclusion criteria rather than inclusion criteria.

5.20   There is an ethical obligation to respect the medical confidentiality of records after death and studies that include deceased workers need to consider this aspect, although the Data Protection Act does not apply to the data of dead people. It is normally considered acceptable to include deceased employees in a records-based study. However, if the protocol involves contacting relatives for further information, for example a case-control study of bladder cancer in the dye industry, it would be important to justify the necessity and to proceed with due sensitivity.

Data security

5.21   Data held for research purposes must be kept just as secure as other occupational health sensitive personal information [see paragraphs 3.18 – 3.24]. Data proliferation of digitally-created and stored files (eg voice recordings of interviews and text files of their transcriptions in qualitative research) is common during the course of a research project as programmes progress from data collection through to analysis and archive and must be planned for.[88] Linkage records are usually destroyed at the end of a study (unless required for later follow-up), but records of destruction should be kept for audit purposes. Data that is retained, which may in certain circumstances be for protracted periods, must be stored under the same secure conditions as when the study was in progress.

Consultation and communication

5.22   Careful consultation with workers or their representatives at the beginning of a study helps to increase participation as well as being good ethical practice. Third party research teams should also involve any local occupational health professional who is best placed to facilitate communication and feedback, and has a key role in establishing trust in the research process. It is important to give subjects a contact name and address for questions about the study, to have a system for logging complaints or questions about the study and to record replies. In both oral and written communications it is important to choose a form and language that can be easily understood. It is particularly important to summarise results and the implications for health in a format suitable for the characteristics of the participants and their relatives. The perception of risk is likely to vary in occupational groups, and this should be taken into account in any communication.

5.23   Effective communication is important not only at the point of recruitment into a study but also throughout the research. In particular there should be a plan for communication of results as part of the study protocol. The group results of research should not be withheld from participants who should be informed preferably before, or at the same time as, wider dissemination to the general public. However it may be important for there to be prior communication to the employer in order that they are in a position to respond to any of the findings in a meaningful way. Where the research topic is sensitive and of interest to the public, there may be pressure from the media to disclose information when the full implications are not clear. In

VIGNETTE 12 : Recruitment and the inadvertent disclosure of sensitive health information during research

A trainee occupational physician, Dr Q, decided as part of her dissertation for Membership of the Faculty (MFOM) to investigate fertility and menstrual irregularities in women who had worked in the semi-conductor industry. She prepared a detailed research protocol, which included a proposal for the invitation to participate in her study, calling for volunteers who *'had previously had a miscarriage or suffered gynaecological problems'*. She proposed that the invitation should take the form of general advertisements, which would be placed on company notice boards in the canteens and rest rooms as well as personal invitations delivered to individual employees with their pay advice slips. On advice from the Research Ethics Committee that the calling notice would be likely to disclose personal information because of the very specific nature of the inclusion criteria, Dr Q re-wrote the invitation to participate, removing the reference to specific women's health issues but restricting the invitation to females. She thought it would subsequently be possible to include targeted questions within her research questionnaire that would address the specific issues she wanted to study. Dr Q successfully recruited over two hundred exposed females from the clean-rooms in the factory as well as a similar number of controls from unexposed workers from a different area.

Issues

Researchers should be aware and sensitive to the fact that any reference to specific inclusion criteria may potentially disclose personal information. Calling/recruitment notices should focus on exclusion criteria rather than inclusion criteria so that individuals can effectively screen themselves out and not volunteer for the research. Where this is not possible then researchers should consider alternative methodology, for example expanding the range of control groups within the study.

For research in the workplace, careful consideration should be given to who communicates with workers about potential participation. There are ethical issues around the interests of different parties and whether employer involvement might be seen as coercion.

Points to consider

What ethical issues would arise if Dr Q wished to write personally to all female workers about her research and to this end requested employers to provide her with a list of employee details?

What legal and ethical issues would arise if:

a) Dr Q requested industry employers to subsequently provide her with information from worker occupational health records?
b) Dr Q was the occupational health provider for the industry and was conducting the study as part of a university postgraduate qualification?

such cases it is particularly important to handle the timing of communication to workers in relation to the media release. Plans for communication of results should, wherever possible, be agreed beforehand with employee representatives. In particularly sensitive situations it might be appropriate to arrange for counselling or discussion (of groups or individuals) to be available. In general, individual results from studies are not disclosed. However, the individual worker should have the right of access to their own results and procedures should be put in place to communicate those appropriately. Consideration should be given to circumstances where research might lead to the identification of undiagnosed illness or unknown workplace risks to workers and arrangements should be put in place for appropriate discussion and counselling.

Research ethics committees

5.24   The role of the research ethics committee (REC) is to provide a review of research proposals which is

independent of those conducting the research and their sponsors. The aim is to protect the dignity, rights, safety and wellbeing of actual or potential research participants, whilst taking accounts of the needs and safety of researchers undertaking good quality research. The REC's review complements researchers' own consideration of the ethical issues raised by their research and helps promote public confidence about the research and conduct of researchers.

5.25   In the UK, RECs are, in the main, governed either by the NHS (Department of Health) or by the universities, although there are a number of independent committees including those of the Health and Safety Executive[89] and the Ministry of Defence.[90]

5.26   The UK Health Departments provide for a National Research Ethics Service (NRES) which sits within the Health Research Authority established in 2011.[91] This Service consists of RECs as well as head offices that co-ordinate the development and management of their operations. A policy document, 'Governance Arrangements for Research Ethics

Committees' (GAfREC)[92] describes the principles, requirements and standards for RECs including their remit, composition, functions, management and accountability. Application to all NHS RECs is via the Integrated Research Application System (IRAS).[93]

5.27   Research ethics committees in the university sector, whilst operating to the same principles as those within the NHS, do not have a central organisation but operate at the level of each university. The principles, requirements and standards to which most university committees subscribe are set out in the Economic and Social Research Council's (ESRC's) Framework for Research Ethics[94] and are broadly compatible with those in GAfREC. Where independent ethical review by a university committee is appropriate, and this may also be a university requirement for indemnity, then researchers are advised to refer to the local university website for their specific arrangements.

5.28   After REC approval has been given, the researcher must not deviate from the protocol without the written prior approval of the REC, except where necessary to protect participants or when changes only involve logistical or administrative aspects that have no ethical implications. However, if an investigator is in any doubt, it is better to seek REC re-approval for any protocol amendments. The principal investigator is required to inform the REC of any adverse events (this most often applies to clinical trials, but it might include a breach of confidentiality or participant complaint) and when an approved project has been completed.

5.29   Similar arrangements for ethical review of research studies are in place in many other countries such as across Europe, North America and Australasia. However, although low- and middle-income countries are increasingly addressing these issues, problems can arise because formal arrangements for ethical approval are not ubiquitous. If research is to be undertaken in occupational populations in countries that are less developed, the researcher should make all reasonable attempts to obtain an independent ethical review and, failing that, comply with the principles of good ethical practice.

Proportionate review

5.30   The notion of proportionate ethical review has been developing over the past decade. Key drivers included the potential workload for RECs and the consequent slow turnaround times for researchers. The initial concept of exempting studies with 'no material ethical issues', has developed into one of 'low risk' or 'minimal risk'. Minimal risk has been clearly defined in this context as meaning 'that the probability and magnitude of harm or discomfort anticipated in the research are not greater in and of themselves than those ordinarily encountered in daily life or during the performance of routine physical or psychological examinations tests'.[95]

5.31   Proportionate ethical review provides for different levels of procedure for projects dependent on an initial evaluation of the risk. This assessment of the risk may be determined by a checklist approach or by a categorisation of specific 'high risk' research. In practice there are a number of systems in place:

- ***Proportionate review based on a checklist approach***
  In NRES research, 'suitable for proportionate review' is determined by the 'No Material Ethical Issues Tool'.[96] This short checklist is completed by the researcher and then submitted for review and approval by a proportionate review sub-committee on behalf of the REC. A number of universities have implemented a checklist which all investigators are required to complete prior to the commencement of their study. This checklist identifies those projects which require a full submission to a REC.

- ***Proportionate review based on professional guidelines***
  Professional guidance in the social sciences suggests proportionate review defined in relation to 'minimal risk'. For example professional guidance from the Government Social Research Unit[97] states that 'projects regarded as presenting 'minimal risk only' do not need to be subjected to formal ethical review' whilst proposals that represent more than minimal risk require greater vigilance with respect to ethical issues throughout their lifespan.
  The ESRC notes that all (ESRC-funded) research must be subject to at least a light touch review which can be handled by a REC sub-committee and can be undertaken using a pre-defined checklist. Where the potential risk of 'substantive' harm to participants and others affected by the proposed research is minimal, this may be all that is necessary. Where a light touch review has confirmed that a research proposal requires full ethics review and approval, this should be carried out by a REC.

- ***Proportionate review based on a template***
  This approach is employed by a number of universities which use it primarily to reduce the number of student applications which would otherwise require full independent review. This is effectively giving approval to a generic research proposal.

Ethics in publication

5.32   It is important that the findings of high quality research are disseminated widely and particularly in occupational health where the evidence base for practice is relatively weak. Care must be taken to avoid publication bias (the tendency for non-publication of results that are negative or which are not in keeping with established paradigms) and to seek balanced publication, by including negative or unusual findings and not exaggerating positive findings. Authors should not pursue, without justification and disclosure, publication of the same or similar results in more than one peer-reviewed journal. Commercial secrecy in the private sector and political embarrassment in the public sector can both be barriers to the dissemination of information. Occupational health professionals are well placed to understand potential sensitivities in their organisation and, whether conducting research themselves or facilitating external researchers, they should ensure that issues are addressed in advance of studies, commencing with (preferably written) agreement about the dissemination of results.

5.33   Journal editors are expected to encourage ethical research through endeavouring to ensure that research they publish has been conducted according to the relevant internationally accepted guidelines. In doing this they will seek assurances that all relevant research has been approved by an appropriate body, for example an independent research ethics committee, where one exists.[98]   Where research has not been independently reviewed then authors should provide evidence that they have considered and met the appropriate ethical standards.   Protecting the confidentiality of individual information obtained in the course of research or professional interactions, for example between occupational health professionals and workers, is of particular concern. It is therefore almost always necessary to obtain written consent for publication from people who might recognise themselves or be identified by others, for example from case reports. It may be possible to publish individual information without express consent if:

(i)   public interest considerations outweigh possible harms;
(ii)   it is impossible to obtain consent; and
(iii)   a reasonable individual would be unlikely to object to publication.

All three criteria must be met and authors should submit a full justification to the editor on submission for publication.

5.34   Occupational health professionals may be invited to give a critical review of funding applications and manuscripts offered for publication. Reviewers should ensure that they are impartial, competent in the subject and that reviews are courteous and as constructive as possible.   Open review, whereby the identity of author and reviewer are declared, is becoming more common. While this has advantages, it is also potentially subject to abuse if an author who receives an adverse review reacts in a way that might disadvantage a referee at a later stage. This is a particular problem where there is a mismatch in seniority or a purchaser/provider relationship might exist. Reviewers must always declare any conflicts of interest (eg financial, material benefit, personal rivalry or collaboration) honestly.   If impartiality is in doubt the invitation to review should be declined.

5.35   The rules of authorship can sometimes give rise to ethical difficulties in publication. Views about authorship of original research papers have changed in recent years. Some leading journals now support the concept of contributorship, encouraging authors to describe their contribution to a study and associated output explicitly. In order to be named as an author, an individual should normally have contributed to the planning, analysis and interpretation of a research study. It is not enough simply to have collected data, or to be in a position of seniority in the research department. Guidance on authorship is given by the International Committee of Medical Journal Editors.[99]

TABLE: Differentiating usual practice in occupational health, research, clinical audit, and service evaluation.

(Adapted from 'Defining Research': National Research Ethics Service, 2009.)

USUAL OCCUPATIONAL HEALTH PRACTICE	RESEARCH	SERVICE EVALUATION*	CLINICAL AUDIT
Designed to investigate ill-health or incidents in a workplace to help in event control and prevention.	Designed to derive generalisable new knowledge through systematic investigation. Will include studies that aim to generate hypotheses as well as studies that aim to test them.	Designed and conducted solely to define or judge current occupational health service delivery.	Designed and conducted to produce information to inform delivery of best occupational healthcare.
Designed to answer: "What is the (likely) cause of this event?"	Designed to characterize populations or to test a hypothesis (quantitative research) or to identify/explore themes following established methodology (qualitative research).	Designed to answer: "What standard does this service achieve in occupational health practice?"	Designed to answer: "Does this service reach a predetermined standard in occupational health practice?"
Systematic, statistical methods may be used.	Addresses clearly defined questions, aims and objectives.	Measures current service without reference to a standard.	Measures against a (gold) standard.
Any management decision is based on clinical best evidence or professional consensus.	May involve evaluating or comparing interventions, particularly new ones (quantitative research) or studying how interventions and relationships are experienced (qualitative research).	Involves an intervention in use only. Management decisions are those of the clinician and worker according to guidance, professional standards and/or worker preference.	Involves an intervention in use only. Management decisions are those of the clinician and worker according to guidance, professional standards and/or worker preference.
May involve administration of interview or questionnaire within the workplace.	Usually involves collecting data that are additional to those for usual practice but may include data collected routinely. May involve treatments, samples or investigations additional to usual practice.	Usually involves analysis of existing data but may include administration of interview or questionnaire.	Usually involves analysis of existing data but may include administration of interview or questionnaire.
May involve a control group to assess risk and identify source of the event but mitigation unaffected.	Study design may involve allocating workers to intervention groups (quantitative research) or use a clearly defined sampling framework underpinned by conceptual or theoretical justifications (qualitative research).	No allocation to intervention: the occupational health professional and worker may have chosen intervention before service evaluation.	No allocation to intervention: the occupational health professional and worker may have chosen intervention before audit.
No randomization.	May involve randomisation.	No randomisation.	No randomisation.
Does not require independent ethical review.	Normally requires independent ethical review by a research ethics committee.	Does not routinely require independent ethical review.	Does not routinely require independent ethical review.

* Service development and quality improvement may fall into this category.

6   FITNESS FOR WORK: THE LEGAL-ETHICAL INTERFACE

Introduction

6.1   Much of occupational health practice is about helping workers and employers navigate the interface between work and health within the constraints of the legal framework. This section looks at a worker's engagement with work across the spectrum from pre-employment considerations, through reasonable adjustments and absence management, to leaving work because of ill-health. The examples used are from UK law to provide a succinct guide for the occupational health professional on the legal parameters around aspects of employment for ethical occupational health practice. It complements and elaborates on issues discussed from an ethical basis in previous sections, particularly Section 3, Information and Section 4, Workplace Health and Wellbeing.

Pre-employment

Health assessment prior to commencing work

6.2   The term pre-employment covers both the period between the worker's job application and the employer's offer of employment, and the period between the job offer and the worker starting work (often called pre-placement). The purpose of pre-employment health assessment is principally to identify those who may need adjustments to the work environment and working practices to allow them to do the job, or to protect them and others against risks arising from their work. In a minority of cases it will be necessary to reject those job applicants whose medical condition or disability renders them unfit.

6.3   According to the law of negligence, the occupational physician owes no duty of care in respect of economic loss to the job applicant pre-employment, though he does owe a duty of care to the employer to whom he reports.[100] He has a duty to take reasonable care with regard to the job applicant's physical welfare,[101] and also owes a duty of confidence and a duty not unlawfully to discriminate against a person with a disability under the Equality Act 2010.

6.4   Asking questions about someone's health is an invasion of that person's privacy which has to be justified under both the Human Rights Act 1998 and the Data Protection Act 1998. The Data Protection Act provides that personal data shall be adequate, relevant and not excessive in relation to the purpose or purposes for which they are processed.[30] The Information Commissioner advises that health questionnaires should be designed and interpreted by health professionals.[102] Madan and Williams[103] found that there was no evidence from the National Health Service to suggest that general health screening for employment is effective and recommended that screening should be confined to criteria identified as being essential for the job. It is for the occupational health professional to advise managers of those criteria, which may differ from job to job. Although lengthy health questionnaires have been in widespread use in recruitment their continued use should now be challenged by health professionals involved in such procedures. Occupational health professionals should ensure that questionnaires ask only relevant questions.

6.5   In addition, individuals should not be expected to reveal clinical details to staff who are not covered by a code of professional ethics imposing a duty of confidence. The advice of the Information Commissioner in Part 4 of the Employment Practices Data Protection Code 2005[102] is that decisions on a worker's suitability for particular work are properly management decisions, but that the interpretation of medical information must be left to a suitably qualified health professional, and that only such persons should have access to medical details. For that reason good ethical practice is that health questionnaires should be processed by qualified medical or nursing staff or, if by others, that the job applicant should be made fully aware of who is to receive the information, and given the option of confining disclosure to a health professional in confidence, for example in a sealed envelope. In the latter case the information should not be made available to human resources or other managers, except with the consent of the worker.

6.6   The anti-discrimination laws enshrined in the Equality Act 2010 prohibit discrimination because of a protected characteristic, that is age, disability, gender reassignment, marriage and civil partnership, pregnancy and maternity, race, religion or belief, sex and sexual orientation, except where the act of discrimination is justified. The law of disability discrimination is the most important for the occupational health professional. The final decision as to whether a worker has a disability within the definition in the Equality Act is for the employment tribunal, not the health professional, but the latter may give an opinion on whether the worker has a physical or mental impairment which has a substantial and long-term adverse effect on his ability to carry out normal day-to-day activities. Long-term means that the impairment has lasted for twelve months, is likely to last for twelve months or is terminal. Cancer, HIV infection and multiple sclerosis are disabilities from diagnosis. Medical conditions should be assessed without medication or prosthesis or other aid (apart from spectacles or contact lenses), for example diabetes without insulin and hearing without a hearing aid. Reference should be made to the official guidance on the definition of disability.[104]

6.7   If the employer is allowed to ask health questions of job applicants before making a job offer it is possible that someone who has a disability may be rejected ostensibly for reasons other than his medical condition, but in fact because of an underlying discriminatory motive. For that reason section 60 of the Equality Act 2010 provides that as a general rule questions about health (which include questions about sickness absence) must not be asked before offering work or, where the employer is not in a position to offer work, before including the job applicant in a pool from which he intends (when in a position to do so) to select a person to whom to offer work. The offer of work may be conditional or unconditional and can be made subject to health clearance, thus permitting health questions to be asked post job offer but pre-employment. If the job applicant is found unsuitable at that stage the conditional offer may be withdrawn, but if he has a disability within the Equality Act he may still make a complaint of disability discrimination to an employment tribunal if he can prove that the employer's reason for rejecting him is related to the disability and cannot be justified, or that the employer has failed to make a reasonable adjustment. The Equality and Human Rights Commission has power to sue an employer which has contravened section 60 in a county court in England and Wales or sheriff court in Scotland. If a disabled job applicant who has been asked health questions pre-job offer and been rejected takes a claim for disability discrimination to an employment tribunal the burden will be on the employer to prove that he has not unlawfully discriminated because of the disability.

1046.8   There are exceptions. The most important are where the employer asks a health question in order to establish whether reasonable adjustments may be needed to an assessment procedure like an interview or written test, or where the question is necessary to establish whether the job applicant will be able to carry out a function that is intrinsic to the work concerned, after reasonable adjustments have been made. Tests of strength, eyesight and hearing for jobs such as the police or fire fighting would fall within this category. Other exceptions are where the job is only open to applicants with certain disabilities (where this is exceptionally permitted, for example where a charity representing people with a disability seeks to recruit a worker with that disability), for diversity monitoring, where positive discrimination is exceptionally allowed, as, for example where an employer guarantees to interview certain disabled job applicants, and for the purpose of vetting applicants for work for reasons of national security.

EXAMPLE 2:

S applies for a job as a scaffolder. On the application form he is asked whether there is any reason why he cannot climb ladders or work at a height, both tasks intrinsic to the job. The employer is entitled to ask this question and, if S discloses that he has difficulty in working at a height, to ask additional questions about whether reasonable adjustments might enable S to do the job. Even if S volunteers that he has epilepsy, and is therefore disabled, the employer can lawfully reject him if a competent risk assessment indicates that such work is hazardous for him, as long as there is no adjustment that can reasonably be made to accommodate him.[105]

6.9   An employer has a positive duty under the Act to make reasonable adjustments to the work or the working environment and to provide auxiliary aids, including auxiliary services, where a job applicant has a disability. Such adjustments should always be considered before recommending that the job applicant is medically unfit for the job.[106] The issue of what is reasonable is for the manager, not occupational health, to decide, and depends on whether the suggested adjustment is practicable, will assist and how much it will cost. Reference should be made to the advisory Code of Practice on Employment published by the Equality and Human Rights Commission.[105] Further information about the legal requirements may be found in standard texts.[9, 107-108]

6.10   Employers   and   occupational   health professionals should not impose blanket exclusions or restrictions on people with a disability simply because of the fact of the disability, since this is direct discrimination which cannot be justified under the Equality Act, unless there is a specific statutory requirement, for example Driver and Vehicle Licensing Agency (DVLA) conditions to obtain a valid driving

EXAMPLE 1:

A construction company asks all job applicants to fill in health questionnaires provided by an occupational health professional when they apply for a job. R applies for a job as a site engineer and discloses in the health questionnaire that he has suffered episodes of depression. R is well qualified and has relevant experience, but he is rejected without an interview. He believes that the true reason is his medical history and claims disability discrimination in an employment tribunal. The employer will have the burden of proving that his disability was not the reason for rejecting him, otherwise he will have to pay compensation to R. It would, however, be permissible for the employer to make offers of jobs conditional on health clearance and then to administer the health questionnaire,[106] though R would still have a claim against the employer if he could prove that he had been unlawfully discriminated against because of a disability.

> **EXAMPLE 3:**
>
> *An employer allows a disabled person to work flexible hours to enable him to have additional breaks to overcome fatigue arising from his disability. This arrangement could also include permitting part-time working or different working hours to avoid the need for travel in the rush hour if this creates a problem related to the impairment. These are likely to be reasonable adjustments.[105]*

licence. Each case should be assessed as an individual, because the effects of a medical condition, for example diabetes and mental illness, can vary from person to person. A job application can be rejected or an employee dismissed because of something arising from the disability, for example a poor attendance record or safety concerns, but only if the employer proves that it is a proportionate means of achieving a legitimate aim.

> **EXAMPLE 4:**
>
> *A residential school for children with severe learning disabilities advertises for a carer. After T is appointed he reveals to his manager that he is infected with HIV. The employer dismisses him because he fears that a child may bite T and the virus be transmitted. Guidance from the UK Panel for Healthcare Workers with Bloodborne Viruses is that there is no evidence of transmission of the virus through biting. This is not direct discrimination, because the employer's reason for dismissing T is the consequence of his infection (the hazard to the children), rather than the infection itself. It is legitimate to take steps to protect the health and safety of the children, but dismissal is not a proportionate response, because there is no evidence that the employment of T creates a real risk therefore the employer is liable for discrimination arising from a disability.[109]*

6.11   Employers should make reasonable adjustments to attendance procedures where a worker is disabled, for example allowing a worker with cancer to take a period of disability leave for treatment and rehabilitation.[105]

6.12   If health screening will include drugs or alcohol tests, employers should advise applicants of this and also whether a positive test will be a bar to employment. They will then have the option to proceed or not on an informed basis [see paragraph 4.32 on drug and alcohol testing].

6.13   Forms seeking consent for access to existing health data such as the entire general practitioner (GP) record should not be used, other than in exceptional cases where it is genuinely necessary. It may be acceptable to ask for consent to ask specific questions of the GP, but such requests will be subject to the Access to Medical Reports Act 1988.

6.14   When reporting to management on the outcome of a pre-employment health assessment applicants should be classified as fit for employment or fit for employment subject to adjustments to the work or the work environment. It is for the employer to determine whether the suggested adjustments are reasonable. It will be exceptional for a person to be classified by occupational health as completely unfit for employment. The duty of reasonable adjustment does not apply where the employer does not know and could not reasonably be expected to know that a person has a disability which is likely to place him at a disadvantage in the workplace. The Equality and Human Rights Commission Code of Practice on Employment 2011 suggests that if an agent or employee, such as an occupational health professional, knows of a disability the employer will not usually be able to claim that they do not know of it, because it will be assumed that the occupational health professional shared it with the employer. However, the Code also states that the Act does not prevent a disabled person keeping a disability confidential from an employer, and in a case involving liability for personal injury the Court of Appeal held that an employer was not deemed to know a job applicant's history of depression which she had disclosed to occupational health but which had not been passed on to management, because she had not given consent for them to be informed.[110] The occupational health professional should explain that, unless consent is given for limited information to be given to the manager in order that adjustments may be proposed, the employer will have no duty to make adjustments. If the disabled person refused to consent to any disclosure this should be documented in the notes.

6.15   Where it is later discovered that a job applicant has not disclosed a particular condition on a pre-employment health questionnaire and information comes to light that would have made a difference to the assessment, for example a medical condition that puts workers or members of the public at serious risk, the occupational health professional should re-assess the risk, taking into account the passage of time. The consent of the individual should be sought to notify the employer of the revised assessment with a clear explanation of the reasons for this. Where consent is refused the occupational health professional will need to decide whether the need to protect third parties overrides his duty of confidence and whether he is entitled to make disclosure without consent. If the new information indicates that the worker may have a disability the professional should undertake the same procedures as he would have done had he been aware of the full facts at the time the worker was applying for the job. Any report to the manager should be presented without gratuitous speculation as to the reason for the original failure to disclose. If the employer asks whether health problems which have later emerged were disclosed on the pre-employment health questionnaire the health professional should reply that the questionnaire is a confidential medical record that will not be disclosed without consent or a court order.[111] The consent of the worker can be sought for release of this information.

6.16   In general there is no duty on a job applicant to volunteer to the employer information about his health, but if asked a specific question, for example, whether he is currently taking any medication prescribed by a doctor, he has a duty to give a truthful reply or be at risk of being held liable for misrepresentation. However, it must be recognised that people without medical training may reply honestly but inaccurately to such a question because they do not fully understand its implications. A job applicant asked: "Do you have a disability?" may honestly answer that he does not because he does not comprehend the complex legal definition of disability. For example a well-controlled insulin dependent diabetic may not understand that the test of disability in the Equality Act assesses him without his insulin and that it is therefore likely that he is classified as disabled.[112]

6.17   Where a worker has obtained a licence from a licensing authority (eg DVLA, Civil Aviation Authority) to perform his work, for example a driver of vehicles on the public highway, there is commonly a statutory duty on the worker to disclose to the licensing authority a health condition which affects his ability to operate safely, and breach of this is a criminal offence. The occupational health professional who becomes aware that a worker is failing to disclose a relevant health condition to a licensing authority, and who concludes that he is thereby creating a risk to others, may reveal confidential medical information to the licensing authority or the employer without consent in the public interest. In addition, where an applicant for employment is a registered medical professional or other health professional there may be an ethical duty to reveal a relevant serious medical condition which may put patients or colleagues at risk, following General Medical Council (GMC) guidance on Good Medical Practice. When considering if a report needs to be made without consent by occupational health to the manager or the professional body, occupational health professionals may wish to discuss the matter in confidence with senior colleagues.[3]

In employment

Duty of care to workers in employment

6.18   Where a worker is in employment the occupational health professional owes a duty to take reasonable care to protect him against risks to his physical or mental health. This may involve advising the worker about hazards or advising the employer about necessary health and safety precautions. In a leading case an occupational physician was held to be negligent in not advising workers or the employer about a carcinogenic substance which created a risk of cancer of the scrotum.[113] Advice should be put into writing and dated.

Specific legislation and standards for fitness for certain occupations

6.19   Some occupational groups have fitness standards laid down in legislation, for example drivers, food handlers and seafarers. There are health and safety laws regulating the employment of pregnant women and children and young workers under 18. Other professionals, such as doctors and nurses, are regulated by their professional organisations. Workers in the public sector, like the police and the fire service, are subject to official guidance from government departments. It goes without saying that legislation is binding and must be applied. However, occupational health professionals should be alert to the duty not to discriminate against persons with a disability in the Equality Act 2010. Each employee or job applicant must be assessed as an individual. Rejection of a worker on vague 'health and safety grounds' will be unlawful unless backed by evidence that there is a specific legislative requirement or that even with reasonable adjustments the worker cannot be safely employed.

> *EXAMPLE 5:*
>
> *V is a lorry driver. He holds a large goods vehicle (LGV) licence. He has recently been diagnosed with insulin dependent diabetes, which means that his licence has been revoked by the DVLA. The employer has no other work for him to do. The employer is entitled to dismiss him because without a licence he cannot lawfully drive his vehicle on the road. However, if there is other work available the employer must not reject him just because of his diabetes. A risk assessment must be performed and reasonable adjustments considered.[105]*

Assessment of fitness to join the pension scheme

6.20   The occupational pension landscape is changing with a declining number of organisations offering defined benefit schemes. Alternative arrangements, such as defined contribution schemes, are less likely to involve occupational health professionals in undertaking pension-related health assessments and are much less likely to require concurrent assessments by the same professional of employment and pensions issues. It will increasingly be unnecessary for a report on whether an applicant is fit for employment to be directed to the employing organisation and a second report on whether he is fit to join the pension scheme to be addressed to the pension trustees. The scope for confusion of role and conflict of interest is therefore diminishing, but nevertheless remains a source of difficulty.

6.21   An individual who is fit for the job, even if only with the application of reasonable adjustments, will normally be fit to join the pension scheme. Under the Equality Act 2010 the employer must not discriminate against a disabled person in the provision of benefits such as pensions and group insurance schemes. However, it may be justifiable to exclude some individuals with a medical condition from access to the full range of benefits provided by an occupational pension scheme. Some pension schemes (for example the police) apply restrictions on access to ill-health retirement benefits. Decisions must be made on a case-by-case basis taking the individual disabled person's circumstances into consideration. Any health declaration must indicate the purpose or purposes for which the information will be used. If information is being used for both pre-employment health assessment and entry to a pension scheme, this should be made clear.

6.22   Where occupational health professionals are requested to provide confidential information to the trustees of a pension scheme the same duty of confidence applies as when they are reporting to a manager. The professional must obtain the worker's consent to write a report to the trustees, and should offer the worker the opportunity of reading the report before it is sent in order that he may be able to point out inaccuracies or withdraw consent if he is unhappy with it. The professional should not change his opinion because of pressure from the worker, but may correct factual errors.

6.23   In some cases the pension trustees have obtained medical reports from doctors responsible for clinical care and have submitted these to the occupational health professional for his assessment. Here the worker has already given consent to the disclosure of confidential data and therefore further consent does not need to be sought.

Attendance and performance management

Certification of sickness absence

6.24   Employees are entitled to the payment of Statutory Sick Pay (SSP) while unable to work through ill-health for a period of up to 28 weeks.[114] No payment is due for the first three days of absence. Many employers supplement this by paying workers their normal basic pay for a period laid down in the contract of employment.

6.25   General practitioners in the National Health Service are required by their contracts to provide certificates of unfitness for work to a patient after an

absence of seven days. Where an employee is absent for fewer than seven days it is common for employers to oblige him to complete a self-certificate. The GP 'fit note', although its ostensible purpose is to certify entitlement to SSP, is taken by many employers and also employment tribunals as evidence that the employee's sickness absence is genuine and of the reason for the absence. The GP may state that the employee is unfit for all work, but may as an alternative state that he is fit for some work. An occupational physician may be asked to advise an employer about whether available work is suitable and whether the employee should be allowed to return. Employers are advised to discuss the matter with the employee and reach agreement. The employer is not under a legal duty to try to find alternative work for the employee unless he has a disability and there is a duty of reasonable adjustment. In a few cases the occupational health professional may disagree with the advice of the GP. Good practice is for the occupational health professional to communicate with the GP, with the employee's consent, as the GP may not have information about the work situation. A few tribunal decisions have held that an employer is entitled to prefer the advice of the occupational physician. Some employers allow the employee to ask for a further opinion from an independent physician in such cases.

EXAMPLE 6:

An employee of a rail company accidentally pricked her finger on a discarded hypodermic needle when clearing rubbish from a carriage. She worked in a safety critical role. She went off sick with depression. On the recommendation of an occupational physician she was assessed by an independent psychiatrist who reported that she was fit to return to work, though she would remain vulnerable to depressive episodes. The occupational physician, however, refused to certify her as fit to return to safety critical work, because her judgment when she was depressed was poor, and this might recur. The manager followed the advice of the occupational physician. A court held that the manager was justified in relying on the advice of the occupational physician.[115]

Assessment of recurrent or prolonged sickness absence

6.26   Control of sickness absence is a management responsibility. The occupational health professional has a role in providing the impartial clinical advice necessary to enable managers to discharge that responsibility in a manner that is fair to the worker and the organisation, and in accordance with their statutory obligations, if any are applicable. This requires objectivity and impartial evidence-based advice.

6.27   As with pre-employment screening the occupational health professional must bear in mind the employer's duty under the Equality Act not to discriminate against the worker because of a protected characteristic like sex, race or disability, and to make reasonable adjustments to assist a worker with a disability to remain at or return to work. Case law indicates that the employer does not have a duty to provide more sick pay to workers with a disability than to his non-disabled workers, unless the reason for their absence is his failure to provide reasonable adjustments,[116-117] but that he should take into account a worker's disability in the application of attendance procedures. Nevertheless, the law does not require an employer to maintain a disabled worker in employment indefinitely, but only for a reasonable time, which depends on the nature of the employment, the degree of disability, the employer's business needs and the medical evidence.[118-120]

6.28 In giving advice to the employer the occupational health professional must base his opinion on relevant medical evidence, which may involve obtaining a report from a GP or treating consultant, with the worker's consent, especially where the worker is at risk of dismissal. In some cases it may be thought advisable to suggest to the employer that a report from an independent expert physician should be obtained, again with consent, about the functional capacity of the worker. It is important for the occupational health professional to state clearly the questions that he wishes the clinician to answer in the letter of referral.

6.29 In cases of intermittent sickness absence of short duration for a variety of different reasons, rather than a lengthy period of absence because of a single health problem, it is important to assess whether there may be an underlying medical condition giving rise to unreliable attendance.

6.30 If a worker refuses to consent to a medical report being disclosed to his manager the occupational health professional should not give such a report, but should inform the worker that the manager will in those circumstances be able to act without medical evidence.[121] Exceptionally, where the worker constitutes a risk to other workers or the general public, the professional can make disclosure without consent, but should first advise the worker of his intentions.[2]

6.31 If in the opinion of the professional the work constitutes a risk to the worker himself, despite the employer's compliance with reasonable standards of health and safety for the bulk of his workforce, for example because of the worker's particular susceptibility to a substance or to stress or vibration, the worker should be given full information about the hazard and advised that it may not be in his best interests to continue in the job. The GMC *Guidance on Confidentiality (2009)* states that a doctor 'should usually abide by a competent adult's refusal to consent to disclosure, even if their decision leaves them, but nobody else, at risk of

serious harm'.[3] Case law indicates that the employer has in general no legal duty to move a worker from a job against his wishes in order to protect him against himself. One judge said that the employer/employee relationship was not one of schoolmaster/pupil.[122] However, in another case a judge said that where there was a serious risk of death or major injury the employer may have a duty to remove the worker from the hazard against his wishes. The example given was of working at heights with epilepsy.[123]

> **EXAMPLE 7:**
>
> W worked in a factory. She developed dermatitis as a result of exposure to an oil to which she was particularly susceptible. The employer tried to find her work in which she did not come into contact with the oil, but she willingly remained working in the factory and her dermatitis became worse. She sued the employer for continuing to employ her in hazardous conditions but it was held that the employer was not liable because she had voluntarily accepted the risk.[122]

6.32 If the worker, having full mental capacity, refuses consent to any information being given to his manager, the occupational health professional should not normally make disclosure unless there is also a risk to others, or there is a serious risk of death or major injury. The professional is advised to make a contemporaneous note of the advice he has given and the worker's response and to keep it in the occupational health file.

Assessment of fitness to attend a disciplinary interview or meeting

6.33 It is frequently the case that a worker who is accused of misconduct or incapability and is made subject to a disciplinary procedure by his manager will go off sick certified by his GP as suffering from stress, and will refuse to attend investigation and disciplinary meetings on the grounds that he is medically unfit to do so. By virtue of the Employment Rights Act 1996, supplemented by advice from the Advisory, Conciliation and Arbitration Service (ACAS),[124] as a general rule it is unfair to penalise an employee without a proper investigation and a meeting at which the employee is able to put his side of the case, accompanied if he wishes by a colleague or trade union representative. The occupational health professional who is requested to assess whether the worker is fit to attend must ask whether he is capable of understanding the case against him and of replying to the charges, either in person or by instructing a representative. If not, he is unfit, but these cases will be rare. It will often be the case that the worker will find the proceedings distressing, but that delaying the process for a prolonged period will be likely to be more damaging to his health, especially his mental health,[3] than continuing with it. The meeting may be held at a neutral venue, and the worker may be permitted to be accompanied by a friend or family member for emotional support. It may be advisable to involve someone other than the worker's immediate manager if there has been a breakdown in the relationship between them which is contributing to his stress. Attempts to contact the worker or his representative by letter or telephone should be documented and kept in the file. The decision whether to go ahead in his absence is for the manager to make, but the occupational health professional must give advice based on his assessment of the situation, taking into account the welfare of the worker but also the need of the employer to reach a conclusion in the interest of the organisation and the other workers.[125] The ACAS guide accepts that a meeting may eventually be held in the worker's absence if all reasonable attempts to facilitate attendance have failed.

Ill-health retirement

6.34   Clarity of role in the mind of the occupational health professional and in the understanding of all with whom they deal is particularly critical when dealing with ill-health retirement cases. There must be a clear separation between the employment and the pension aspects of the case. In larger schemes this is increasingly achieved through a physical separation of the functions but smaller schemes may have to rely on the employer's medical adviser as the only source of competent advice on specific health-related employment issues. In this latter case, occupational physicians must be assiduous in acting, and being seen to act, impartially. Occupational health professionals advising pension schemes must remember their duties to the trustees of the scheme; this adds the potential for even greater complexity than the dual responsibility to employer and employee that is common in occupational health.

6.35   Ill-health retirement is often viewed by employees and managers alike as an alternative to resignation, redundancy or dismissal. Tribunals have held that, where the prognosis about a worker's medical condition is uncertain, the employer should consider whether the employee might qualify for ill-health retirement or whether he should remain in employment while further medical advice is sought before making the decision to dismiss.[126] Even if the worker has applied for ill-health retirement benefits the employer must ensure that employment decisions are made fairly and in accordance with both the organisation's internal procedures and relevant legislation such as the Employment Rights Act 1996 and the Equality Act 2010. Only when these aspects of the case have been properly dealt with should attention shift to eligibility for ill-health retirement benefits.

6.36   Eligibility for an early or enhanced pension because of ill-health is dependent on the scheme member meeting various criteria as set out in the rules of the scheme. Criteria vary between schemes. In the public sector some pension schemes are laid down in statutory regulations and decisions are susceptible to judicial review. It is essential that professionals are aware of the wording of the scheme in question and official guidance and case law that has interpreted its meaning. There is no substitute for examining the words of the regulations.

6.37   The optimum means of determining whether an individual is likely to meet the criteria for ill-health retirement will necessarily vary on a case-by-case basis. However, it will be usual for evidence to include an assessment of capability matched to the requirements of the job, as well as objective medical evidence about the illness or injury which allows the formulation of a diagnosis and prognosis. In most cases sufficient objective medical evidence can be gleaned from the worker's occupational health records and/or his general practitioner records, but, where this is deficient, it may be necessary to commission independent examinations and/or investigations. When requesting reports from others it should be made clear that advice is sought only on the worker's medical condition, their functional abilities and the prognosis, not on the possible effects on their employment or their entitlement to a pension.

6.38   Advice on eligibility for ill-health retirement should only be given by occupational health professionals who have suitable and sufficient knowledge of the job and the working environment, because it is usually necessary to assess whether the worker is unfit to perform his normal work as well as whether he is incapable of all work. Many pension schemes require their medical advisers to have a qualification in occupational medicine and some larger schemes operate within a quality accreditation environment with written guidelines on application of the criteria and audit of decisions. This represents good practice. All ill-health retirement processes should have a complaints procedure and an appeals mechanism. Initial assessments and assessments at the appeal stage may be undertaken on the basis of either a physical consultation or as a 'papers only' process. Neither is inherently superior from an ethical standpoint. A physical consultation may convey the perception of greater autonomy for the individual but also runs the risk of blurring the boundaries with a therapeutic relationship (which it manifestly is not). Appeal assessments are more likely to be conducted on a 'papers only' basis to try to ensure consistency and because further examination rarely provides new objective evidence.

REFERENCES

(All web addresses below accessed 22 November 2012)

1   *Equality Act 2010.*
     http://www.legislation.gov.uk/ukpga/2010/15/contents

2   General Medical Council. *Consent: patients and doctors making decisions together.* London: GMC, June 2008.
     http://www.gmc-uk.org/static/documents/content/Consent_-_English_0911.pdf

3   General Medical Council. *Confidentiality.* London: GMC, October 2009.
     http://www.gmc-uk.org/static/documents/content/Confidentiality_0910.pdf

4   General Medical Council. *Confidentiality: disclosing information for insurance, employment and similar
     purposes.* London: GMC, September 2009.
     http://www.gmc-uk.org/Confidentiality_disclosing_info_insurance_2009.pdf_27493823.pdf

5   Faculty of Occupational Medicine, Royal College of Physicians of London. *Good occupational medical
     practice.* London: FOM, August 2010.
     http://www.fom.ac.uk/wp-content/uploads/p_gomp2010.pdf

6   Faculty of Occupational Medicine, Royal College of Physicians of London. *Occupational health service
     standards for accreditation.* London: FOM, January 2010.
     http://www.fom.ac.uk/wp-content/uploads/standardsjan2010.pdf and
     http://www.seqohs.org/DocumentStore/fom_seqohs.pdf

7   Beauchamp TL and Childress JF. *Principles of biomedical ethics.* 6th edition. Oxford: Oxford University Press,
     2009.

8   International Commission on Occupational Health. *International code of ethics for occupational health
     professionals.* Singapore: ICOH, 2002.
     http://www.icohweb.org/heritage/pdf/code_ethics_2002.pdf

9   Kloss D. *Occupational health law.* 5th edition. Wiley-Blackwell, 2010

10   Department of Health. *Clinical governance.*
     http://webarchive.nationalarchives.gov.uk/+/www.dh.gov.uk/en/Publichealth/Patientsafety/
     Clinicalgovernance/index.htm

11   Financial Reporting Council. *The UK Corporate Governance Code.* London: FRC, September 2012.
     http://www.frc.org.uk/getattachment/a7f0aa3a-57dd-4341-b3e8-ffa99899e154/UK-Corporate-Governance-
     Code-September-2012.aspx

12   *Sarbanes-Oxley Act of 2002. Public Law 107-204.*
     http://www.gpo.gov/fdsys/pkg/PLAW-107publ204/html/PLAW-107publ204.htm

13   Nursing & Midwifery Council. *The code: Standards of conduct, performance and ethics for nurses and
     midwives.* London: NMC, May 2008.
     http://www.nmc-uk.org/Documents/Standards/The-code-A4-20100406.pdf

14   *Access to Medical Reports Act 1988.*
     http://www.legislation.gov.uk/ukpga/1988/28/contents

15   *Health and Safety at Work Act 1974.*
     http://www.legislation.gov.uk/ukpga/1974/37 contents

16   *The Safety Representatives & Safety Committees Regulations 1977.*
     http://www.legislation.gov.uk/uksi/1977/500/contents/made

17   *The Health & Safety (Consultation with Employees) Regulations 1996.*
        http://www.legislation.gov.uk/uksi/1996/1513/contents/made

18   General Medical Council. *Good medical practice.* London: GMC, November 2006, updated March 2009.
        http://www.gmc-uk.org/static/documents/content/GMP_0910.pdf

19   *Public Interest Disclosure Act 1998.*
        http://www.legislation.gov.uk/ukpga/1998/23/contents

20   General Medical Council. *Good medical practice: Probity: providing and publishing information about your
        services.* London: GMC, November 2006, updated March 2009.
        http://www.gmc-uk.org/guidance/good_medical_practice/probity_information_about_services.asp

21   Faculty of Occupational Medicine. *An employer's guide to engaging an occupational health physician.*
        London: FOM, April 2010.
        http://www.fom.ac.uk/wp-content/uploads/empopguid.pdf

22   Nursing and Midwifery Council. *Specialist community public health nursing.*
        http://www.nmc-uk.org/Nurses-and-midwives/Regulation-in-practice/Specialist-community-public-health-
        nursing/

23   British Psychological Society. *Becoming an occupational psychologist.*
        http://www.bps.org.uk/careers-education-training/how-become-psychologist/types-psychologists/
        becoming-occupational-psychol

24   Ministry of Justice. *Bribery Act 2010 Guidance.*
        http://www.justice.gov.uk/downloads/legislation/bribery-act-2010-guidance.pdf

25   *The Transfer of Undertakings (Protection of Employment) Regulations 2006.*
        http://www.legislation.gov.uk/uksi/2006/246/contents/made

26   *Data Protection Act 1998.*
        http://www.legislation.gov.uk/ukpga/1998/29/contents

27   *Access to Health Records Act 1990.*
        http://www.legislation.gov.uk/ukpga/1990/23/contents
        http://webarchive.nationalarchives.gov.uk/+/www.dh.gov.uk/en/Managingyourorganisation/
        Informationpolicy/Patientconfidentialityandcaldicottguardians/DH_4084411

28   Council of Europe. *European Convention on Human Rights.*
        http://conventions.coe.int/treaty/en/treaties/html/005.htm

29   *Human Rights Act 1998*
        http://www.legislation.gov.uk/ukpga/1998/42/contents

30   *Data Protection Act 1998: Data protection principles*
        http://www.legislation.gov.uk/ukpga/1998/29/schedule/1

31   British Medical Association. *Social media use: practical and ethical guidance for doctors and medical students.*
        BMA: London, 2012.
        http://bma.org.uk/-/media/Files/PDFs/Practical%20advice%20at%20work/Ethics/socialmediaguidance.pdf

32   *The Control of Substances Hazardous to Health Regulations 2002.*
        http://www.legislation.gov.uk/uksi/2002/2677/contents/made

33   *The Ionising Radiations Regulations 1999.*
        http://www.legislation.gov.uk/uksi/1999/3232/contents/made

34   *Mental Capacity Act 2005.*
        http://www.legislation.gov.uk/ukpga/2005/9/contents

35   General Medical Council. *Confidentiality: Disclosing information with consent.* London: GMC, November
        2006, updated March 2009.
        http://www.gmc-uk.org/guidance/ethical_guidance/confidentiality_24_35_disclosing_information_with_
        consent.asp

36   *Human Tissue Act 2004.*
        http://www.legislation.gov.uk/ukpga/2004/30/contents

37   General Medical Council. *Good Medical Practice: Confidentiality – relevant fitness to practise cases.* London:
        GMC, November 2006, updated March 2009.
        http://www.gmc-uk.org/ftp_case_137.pdf_25416447.pdf

38   General Medical Council. *Making and using audio visual recordings of patients.* London: GMC, April 2011.
        http://www.gmc-uk.org/static/documents/content/Making_and_using_visual_and_audio_recordings_of_
        patients_2011.pdf

39   London Borough of Hammersmith and Fulham v Farnsworth [2000] IRLR 691.

40   *The Management of Health and Safety at Work Regulations 1999.*
        http://www.legislation.gov.uk/uksi/1999/3242/contents/made

41   *The Control of Noise at Work Regulations 2005.*
        http://www.legislation.gov.uk/uksi/2005/1643/contents/made

42   *The Control of Vibration at Work Regulations 2005.*
        http://www.legislation.gov.uk/uksi/2005/1093/contents/made

43   *The Control of Lead at Work Regulations 2002.*
        http://www.legislation.gov.uk/uksi/2002/2676/contents/made

44   *The Control of Asbestos Regulations 2006.*
        http://www.legislation.gov.uk/uksi/2006/2739/contents/made

45   *The Diving at Work Regulations 1997.*
        http://www.legislation.gov.uk/uksi/1997/2776/contents/made

46   *The Work in Compressed Air Regulations 1996.*
        http://www.legislation.gov.uk/uksi/1996/1656/contents/made

47   British Medical Association. *Confidentiality and health records. Consent forms for England and Wales and for
        Scotland.*
        http://bma.org.uk/practical-support-at-work/ethics/confidentiality-and-health-records

48   The Police and Criminal Evidence Act 1984 (Codes of Practice) (Revisions to Codes E and F) Order 2010.
        http://www.legislation.gov.uk/uksi/2010/1108/contents/made

49   *Public Health (Control of Diseases) Act 1984.*
        http://www.legislation.gov.uk/ukpga/1984/22/contents

50   *Medical Act 1983.*
        http://www.legislation.gov.uk/ukpga/1983/54/contents
        http://www.gmc-uk.org/about/legislation/medical_act.asp

51   *National Health Service Act 2006.*
        http://www.legislation.gov.uk/ukpga/2006/41/contents

52   National Information Governance Board for Health and Social Care at
      http://www.nigb.nhs.uk/

53   World Health Organisation. *Mental health: a state of well-being.* October 2011
      http://www.who.int/features/factfiles/mental_health/en/index.html

54   General Medical Council. *Raising and acting on concerns about patient safety.* London: GMC, January 2012.
      http://www.gmc-uk.org/Raising_and_acting_on_concerns_about_patient_safety_FINAL.pdf_47223556.pdf

55   Health and Safety Executive. *Line manager competency tool.*
      http://www.hse.gov.uk/stress/mcit.htm

56   Kieselbach, T et al. *Health in restructuring.* Mering: Rainer Hampp Verlag, 2010.
      http://www.workinglives.org/londonmet/fms/MRSite/Research/wlri/WORKS/HIRES%20New%20engl%20
      FR%20FIN.pdf

57   World Health Organisation. *Global status report on non-communicable diseases.* 2010.
      http://www.who.int/nmh/en/
      http://www.who.int/nmh/publications/ncd_report_full_en.pdf

58   World Economic Forum. *Workplace Wellness Alliance.*
      http://www.weforum.org/issues/workplace-wellness-alliance

59   National Institute for Health and Clinical Excellence (NICE). *Public Health Guidance 5: Workplace interventions to promote smoking cessation.* London: April 2007.
      http://guidance.nice.org.uk/PH5

60   National Institute for Health and Clinical Excellence (NICE). *Public Health Guidance 13: Promoting physical activity in the workplace.* London: May 2008.
      http://guidance.nice.org.uk/PH13

61   National Institute for Health and Clinical Excellence (NICE). *Public Health Guidance 22. Promoting mental wellbeing at work.* London: November 2009.
      http://guidance.nice.org.uk/PH22

62   British Medical Association. *The Occupational Physician – guidance for specialists and others practising occupational health.* BMA: July 2011.
      http://www.mrc.ac.uk/consumption/idcplg?IdcService=GET_FILE&dID=6233&dDocName=MRC002452&all
      owInterrupt=1

63   *Equality Act 2010 – Section 60.*
      http://www.legislation.gov.uk/ukpga/2010/15/section/60

64   Department of Health. *Health clearance for tuberculosis, hepatitis B, hepatitis C and HIV: New healthcare workers.* London: DH; March 2007.
      http://www.dh.gov.uk/prod_consum_dh/groups/dh_digitalassets/@dh/@en/documents/digitalasset/
      dh_074981.pdf

65   Department of Health. *HIV infected healthcare workers: Guidance on management and patient notification.* London: DH; July 2005. (Under consultation December 2011-March 2012).
      http://www.dh.gov.uk/prod_consum_dh/groups/dh_digitalassets/@dh/@en/documents/digitalasset/
      dh_4116416.pdf

66   Department of Health. *Hepatitis B infected health care workers: Guidance on implementation of health service circular 2000/020.* London: DH, June 2000.
      http://www.dh.gov.uk/prod_consum_dh/groups/dh_digitalassets/@dh/@en/documents/digitalasset/
      dh_4057538.pdf

67   Department of Health. *Hepatitis B infected healthcare workers and antiviral therapy.* London: DH, March 2007.
        http://www.dh.gov.uk/prod_consum_dh/groups/dh_digitalassets/documents/digitalasset/dh_073133.pdf

68   Department of Health. *Hepatitis C infected health care workers.* London: DH, August 2002.
        http://www.dh.gov.uk/prod_consum_dh/groups/dh_digitalassets/@dh/@en/documents/digitalasset/dh_4059544.pdf

69   UK National Screening Committee. UK Screening Portal. *What is screening?*
        http://www.screening.nhs.uk/screening

70   UK National Screening Committee. UK Screening Portal. *Programme appraisal criteria.*
        http://www.screening.nhs.uk/criteria

71   Wilson JMG, Jungner G. *Principles and practice of screening for disease.* Public Health Paper Number 34. Geneva: WHO, 1968.

72   Faculty of Occupational Medicine, Royal College of Physicians of London. *Guidance on alcohol and drug misuse in the workplace.* London: FOM, 2006.

73   McCann M, Harker Burnhams N, Albertyn C and Bhoola U. *Alcohol, drugs and employment.* 2nd edition. South Africa: Juta, 2011.

74   Human Genetics Commission. *Genetics and employment.*
        http://www.hgc.gov.uk/Client/Content.asp?ContentId=123

75   MacDonald C & Williams-Jones B. Ethics and genetics: susceptibility testing in the workplace. *Journal of Business Ethics* 2002; 35(3): 235-241.
        http://www.biotechethics.ca/wgt/index.html

76   European Commission. *European textbook on ethics in research.* Luxembourg: Publications Office of the European Union, 2010.
        http://ec.europa.eu/research/science-society/document_library/pdf_06/textbook-on-ethics-report_en.pdf

77   Royal College of Physicians. *Guidelines on the practice of ethics committees in medical research with human participants 4th edition.* London: RCP, 2007.

78   Differentiating research, audit and service evaluation/development: a guide from United Bristol Healthcare NHS Trust. 1995.

79   Wade DT. Ethics, audit, and research: all shades of grey. *BMJ* 2005; 330: 468-71.

80   Berdon V. *Codes of medical and human experimentation ethics.* Bloomington: Poynter Centre, 2002. Quoted in Pimple KD (editor). Research Ethics. xv. Ashgate Publishing Ltd, 2008.

81   World Medical Association. *Declaration of Helsinki - Ethical principles for medical research involving human subjects.* June 1964, as amended October 2008.
        http://www.wma.net/en/30publications/10policies/b3/

82   Emanuel EJ, Wendler D and Grady C. What makes clinical research ethical? *JAMA* 2000; 283: 2701-2711.

83   Rothstein MA. Ethical guidelines for medical research on workers. *J Occup Environ Med* 2000; 42: 1166-1171.

84   Rose SL, Pietri CE. Workers as research subjects: a vulnerable population. *J Occup Environ Med* 2002; 44: 801-805.

85   National Research Ethics Service. *Information sheets and consent forms: guidance for researchers and reviewers.* NRES: 2011.
        http://www.nres.nhs.uk/EasysiteWeb/getresource.axd?AssetID=338&type=full&servicetype=Attachment

86   Department of Health. *NHS Confidentiality Code of Practice.* London: DH, 2003.
      http://webarchive.nationalarchives.gov.uk/ı /www.dh.gov.uk/en/Managingyourorganisation/
      Informationpolicy/Patientconfidentialityandcaldicottguardians/DH_4100550

87   Medical Research Council. *Personal information in medical research.* London: MRC, 2000 (addition 2003).
      http://www.mrc.ac.uk/Utilities/Documentrecord/index.htm?d=MRC002452

88   Aldridge J, Medina J, Ralphs R. The problem of proliferation: guidelines for improving the security of
      qualitative data in a digital age. *Res Ethics Rev* 2010; 6: 3-9.

89   Health and Safety Executive Research ethics committee at
      http://www.hse.gov.uk/research/ethics/index.htm

90   Ministry of Defence Research ethics committees at
      http://www.science.mod.uk/Engagement/modrec/modrec.aspx

91   National Research Ethics Service at
      http://www.nres.nhs.uk/

92   Department of Health. *Governance arrangements for research ethics committees: a harmonised edition.*
      London: DH, 2011.
      http://www.dh.gov.uk/en/Publicationsandstatistics/Publications/PublicationsPolicyAndGuidance/
      DH_126474

93   Integrated Research Application System at
      https://www.myresearchproject.org.uk/

94   Economic and Social Research Council. *Framework for research ethics.* ESRC, 2010 (revised 2012).
      http://www.esrc.ac.uk/about-esrc/information/research-ethics.aspx

95   Code of Federal Regulations 45 CFR 46.102(h)(i). *The Regulatory definition of minimal risk.* NIH, 2005
      http://www.hhs.gov/ohrp/humansubjects/guidance/45cfr46.html#46.102

96   National Research Ethics Service. *No Material Ethics Issue tool.* August 2009
      http://www.nres.nhs.uk/applications/proportionate-review/

97   Government Social Research Unit. *Ethical assurance for social research in Government.* London: HM Treasury,
      2005.
      http://www.civilservice.gov.uk/wp-content/uploads/2011/09/ethics_guidance_tcm6-5782.pdf

98   Committee on Publication Ethics. *Code of conduct and best practice guidelines for journal editors.* 2011.
       http://publicationethics.org/files/Code_of_conduct_for_journal_editors_0.pdf

99   International Committee of Medical Journal Editors. *Uniform requirements for manuscripts submitted to
      biomedical journals: ethical considerations in the conduct and reporting of research: authorship and
      contributorship.*
      http://www.icmje.org/ethical_1author.html

100   Kapfunde v Abbey National [1998] IRLR 583

101   R v Croydon Health Authority [1997] Lloyds Med Rep 44

102   Information Commissioner's Office. *Data Protection – The Employment Practices Code.* 2005.
      http://www.ico.gov.uk/upload/documents/library/data_protection/practical_application/ico_suppgdnce.pdf

103   Madan I and Williams S. *A review of pre-employment health screening of NHS staff.* London: TSO, 2010.
      http://www.nhshealthatwork.co.uk/images/library/files/Clinical%20excellence/Pre-employment_for_web_
      final_10.6.10.pdf

104   Office for Disability Issues. *Equality Act 2010. Guidance on matters to be taken into account in determining questions relating to the definition of disability.* SI 2011/1159.
http://odi.dwp.gov.uk/docs/wor/new/ea-guide.pdf

105   Equality and Human Rights Commission: *Code of Practice on Employment.*
http://www.equalityhumanrights.com/uploaded_files/EqualityAct/employercode.pdf

106   *Equality Act 2010: section 20 and schedule 8*
http://www.legislation.gov.uk/ukpga/2010/15/section/20
http://www.legislation.gov.uk/ukpga/2010/15/schedule/8/paragraph/20

107   Lewis J and Thornbory G. *Employment law and occupational health.* 2nd edition. Oxford: Wiley-Blackwell, 2011.

108   Kloss D and Ballard J. *Discrimination law and occupational health practice.* London: The At Work Partnership, 2012

109   High Quality Lifestyles v Watts [2006] IRLR 850

110   Hartman v South Essex Mental Health and Community Care NHS Trust [2005] IRLR 293

111   Cheltenham Borough Council v Laird [2009] IRLR 621

112   *Equality Act 2010 - Schedule 1(5).*
http://www.legislation.gov.uk/ukpga/2010/15/schedule/1

113   Stokes v GKN (Nuts and Bolts) Ltd [1968] 1 WLR 1776

114   *The statutory Sick Pay (Medical Evidence) Regulations (as amended) (1985).* SI 1985/1604.
http://www.legislation.gov.uk/uksi/1985/1604/contents/made

115   Heathrow Express Operating Co Ltd v Jenkins [2007] All ER (D) 144

116   O'Hanlon v Commissioners for HMRC [2007] IRLR 404;

117   Meikle v Nottinghamshire CC [2004] IRLR 703

118   First Manchester Ltd v Kennedy [2005] UKEAT/0818/04

119   Jeffries v BP Tanker Co Ltd [1974] IRLR 260

120   Royal Liverpool Children's NHS Trust v Dunsby [2006] IRLR 351

121   O'Donoghue v Elmbridge Housing Trust [2004] EWCA Civ 939

122   Withers v Perry Chain Co Ltd [1961] 3 All ER 676

123   Coxall v Goodyear (GB) Ltd [2002] IRLR 742

124   ACAS. *Code of Practice 1: Disciplinary and grievance procedures.* London: TSO, April 2009.
http://www.acas.org.uk/media/pdf/k/b/Acas_Code_of_Practice_1_on_disciplinary_and_grievance_
procedures-accessible-version-Jul-2012.pdf

125   ACAS. *Discipline and grievances at work – the ACAS guide.* London: TSO; April 2011.
http://www.acas.org.uk/media/pdf/s/o/Acas-Guide-on-discipline-and-grievances_at_work_(April_11)-
accessible-version-may-2012.pdf

126   First West Yorkshire Ltd v Haigh [2008] IRLR 182

INDEX

absenteeism 4.3
> *see also* sickness absence

Access to Health Records Act 1990 3.1, 3.57
Access to Medical Reports Act 1988 2.14, 3.1, 3.58, 6.13
accreditation 2.33
adjustments to working conditions 4.41–4.42, 6.9
advertising 2.32
Advisory, Conciliation and Arbitration Service (ACAS) 6.33
alcohol, testing for 4.32, 6.12
American College of Occupational and Environmental Medicine 2.28
anonymised data 2.11, 3.71–3.72, 5.16–5.17
audit 2.28, 3.12
auditors, disclosure of information to 3.70
autonomy 1.13, 1.14, 1.16, 3.2, 4.8, 4.23

beneficence 1.13, 1.17, 2.22, 4.4, 4.24
biological monitoring 4.30–4.31
biomedical ethics *see* ethics
Bribery Act (2010) 2.34
British Medical Association 2.38, 3.16, 4.11
British Occupational Health Research Foundation 2.28
business ethics 2.32, 2.35

capacity 3.40
Civil Aviation Authority 6.17
clients *see* patients
clinical colleagues 2.9–2.10
clinical governance *see* governance
clinical information, disclosure *see* disclosure
communicable diseases 3.81
communication 5.22–5.23
company values 2.3–2.4
competence
> of occupational health professionals 2.33
> of patients to make decisions 1.16

competitive tender 2.34–2.35
confidential information, disclosure of 2.9
confidentiality 1.5, 1.14, 2.11, 2.19, 3.1, 3.5–3.7
> ethical and legal duties 3.3, 3.7
> in research 5.16–5.20

conflicting advice 4.43
conflicts of interest 2.24
consent 1.5, 3.37–3.39
> express 3.37
> human tissue samples 3.42
> implied 3.37
> oral 3.44
> for preparation of occupational health report 2.14, 3.43–3.50
> for research 5.12–5.15
> to seek a report from other clinicians 2.14
> for treatment 1.16, 3.41
> withdrawal of 3.50

consultations, recording of 3.51
continuing professional development 2.29
contracted services 2.38
contracts 2.38

ACKNOWLEDGEMENTS

The Faculty of Occupational Medicine would like to thank the numerous individuals involved in the preparation of this document:

- first and foremost the **Faculty Ethics Committee**; all members of the Committee participated in the writing and editorial process; Paul Litchfield and Naomi Brecker edited the guidance, and Frances Quinn prepared the document for publication;
- Faculty members who volunteered to join a **consultative group** to offer comments on specific issues, draft text for the evolving guidance and comment on drafts of the various sections;
- the wider **stakeholder community** consulted to ensure that their concerns and views were reflected in the new guidance.

The individuals and organisations are listed below.

The work of all those who contributed to previous editions is gratefully acknowledged also.

Members of the Faculty Ethics Committee

Paul Litchfield OBE OStJ MSc FRCP FFOM   Chair
Naomi Brecker MA FFPH MFOM   Secretary
Graham Bell MSc FRCP FFOM
Sarah Cave MSc RN SPOHN MIOSH
John Challenor FRCP FFOM
Peter Graham BSc PhD Hon FFOM
Barbara Harrison BSc MSc CMIOSH MFOH
Louise Holden MBA MMedSci FFOM
Sue Hunt MB BS MFOM DTM&H
Bob Jefferson BSc FFOM CMIOSH
Diana Kloss MBE LLB LLM Barrister Hon FFOM
Sarah Page RGN BSc PGDip
Berend Rah MD PhD DOccMed
Roger Rawbone MB BS MA MD Hon FFOM
Simon Sheard MMedSci FRCP FFOM FFSEM DAvMed
Lizzie Wood MBA RN ONC NDN SPCPHN PGDip

Secretariat: Frances Quinn

Members of the consultative group

Paul Baker, John Ballard, Lisa Birrell, Peter Graham, David Jenkins, Ian Lambert, Paul Lian, Karen Nightingale, Shritti Pattani, Chris Sharp, Jacques Tamin, Michael Vaughan, Liz Wright.

Stakeholder organisations

Association of British Insurers

Association of Chartered Physiotherapists in Occupational Health and Ergonomics

Association of Insurance and Risk Managers in Industry and Commerce (UK)

Association of Occupational Health Nurse Practitioners (UK)

Association of NHS Occupational Health Nurses

Association of National Health Occupational Physicians

Association of Local Authority Medical Advisors

Association of Railway Industry Occupational Health Practitioners

British Association of Occupational Therapists and College of Occupational Therapists

British Medical Association

British Occupational Hygiene Society

British Psychological Society

Chartered Institute of Environmental Health

Chartered Institute of Personnel and Development

Chartered Society of Physiotherapy

Confederation of British Industry

Commercial Occupational Health Providers Association

Department of Health, England

Department of Health, Social Services and Public Safety, Northern Ireland

Scottish Government Health Directorate

Welsh Assembly Government

Department for Work and Pensions

EEF The Manufacturers' organisation

Faculty of Public Health

Faculty of Sport and Exercise Medicine

General Medical Council

Health and Safety Executive

Institution of Occupational Safety and Health

National Director for Health and Work

Nursing and Midwifery Council

Royal College of Nursing - Public Health Forum

Royal College of General Practitioners

Royal College of Physicians (London) - Ethical Issues in Medicine Committee

Royal College of Psychiatrists

Society of Occupational Medicine

Trades Union Congress